THE HEALING POWERS OF
CHELATION THERAPY

Unclog Your Arteries
An Alternative to
Bypass Surgery

by

John Parks Trowbridge, M.D.
and
Morton Walker, D.P.M.

NEW WAY OF LIFE, Inc.
484 High Ridge Road
Stamford, Connecticut 06905

A LIFE ENHANCEMENT BOOK

i

Published by
NEW WAY OF LIFE, Inc.
484 High Ridge Road
Stamford, Connecticut 06905 U.S.A.
(203) 322-1551 or (203) 323-2808

Editor Morton Walker, D.P.M.

Manufactured in the United States of America.

Library of Congress Cataloging in Publication Data
Library of Congress New Card Number 88-92507
Trowbridge, John Parks.
    Chelation therapy

    1.   Atherosclerosis—Chemotherapy.   2.   Chelation therapy.
I. Walker, Morton.   II. Title. [DNLM: 1. Arterial Occlusive Diseases—drug therapy—popular works. 2. Blood Circulation—drug effects—popular works. 3. Chelating Agents —therapeutic use—popular works. WG 113 T863r]
RC692.T76 1985 616.1'3061 (Previously Published by Devin-Adair, Publishers, Old Library of Congress Catalog Card Number 84-28741)
New ISBN 0-945498-01-2
(Previously Published by Devin-Adair, Publishers, Old ISBN 0-8159-5228-7)

DISCLAIMER

This book has been written and published strictly for informational purposes. In no way should it be used as a substitute for your own physician's advice.

While John Parks Trowbridge, M.D. and Morton Walker, D.P.M., are collaborating here as coauthors, Dr. Trowbridge is the physician expert on chelation therapy and Dr. Walker is the medical journalist reporting on such health care information.

You should not consider educational material in the book to be the practice of medicine, although almost all the facts have come from the files, publications, and personal interviews of informed physicians who diagnose and treat cardiovascular diseases and/or their patients who have suffered from such conditions.

If you, as a potential user of knowledge received from these pages, require opinions, diagnoses, treatments, therapeutic advice, correction of your lifestyle, or any other aid relating to your health or to chelation therapy, it is recommended that you consult either Dr. Trowbridge, the other physicians contributing to this book or a chelating physician trained by the American Board of Chelation Therapy.

These statements are to be considered disclaimers of responsibility for anything published here. The coauthors provide the information in this book with the understanding that you may act on it at your own risk and also with full knowledge that health professionals should first be consulted and that their specific advice for you should be considered before anything read here.

CONTENTS

What is Chelation Therapy?

Chelation therapy is the administration, under the supervision of a physician, of a protein-like substance, combined with other nutrients, into a vein of your body. It is a process that takes several hours, so that the nutrients slowly circulate through the 60,000 miles of blood vessels that feed your body's organs, tissues, and cells. Chelation therapy, by ridding your body of potentially deadly poisons, can, more than any other therapeutic agent, give you the gift of longer life.

Chelation is a derivitive of the Greek word *chele*, meaning *claw*, as that of a lobster or crab. The chelate substance, particularly the protein (a man-made amino acid), grasps certain minerals, usually metal atoms such as lead, mercury, cadmium or others with two available bonds, or valences. The metal atom becomes locked in by the encircling amino acid, which, since it does not combine with any part of the human body, has nowhere to go—except out of the body.

Most of it passes out through the kidneys as part of the urine, during the first 24 hours following the administration of chelation therapy. And with the amino acid travels the captured metallic ions that may very well have been producing toxic effects in your body.

By the chelation of toxins from the cells, the life of those cells has been extended. Your body has been rid of much accumulated devastation from, for example, metallic pollutants you've eaten, destructive free radicals produced by food additives, chemicals and radiation, and assorted foreign elements that cause cellular break-down.

Who Is a Candidate for Chelation Therapy?

At 70 years old, John Parks Trowbridge, Sr., is retired from the U.S. Air Force and resides in Hollister, California. "Jack"—to those who know him—impresses you by the deep resonance of his voice, the erect manner in which he carries himself, and the vigor of his movements. But Jack Trowbridge wasn't always so vigorous.

In 1975, an alert physician who was giving him a routine physical examination discovered that Jack had an aortic aneurysm. This is a balloon-like swelling in the wall of the body's main artery, which damages the vessel's muscular coat as the result of degeneration. This weakness is apt to cause tearing in the lining of the aorta, which allows blood to enter the artery's wall and track along the muscular coat. The danger is that this dissecting aneurysm may rupture or may compress smaller blood vessels arising from the aorta and produce infarction (localized death) in the organs they supply.

"The upshot of the discovery of my aneurysm was a quick trip to the hospital to get a surgical repair," said Mr. Trowbridge. "The surgeons split me from the rib bones down and patched a plastic tube into my abdominal aorta, the major artery running along my backbone to divide into two vessels for feeding the legs. Also, the doctors found that I was having generalized arterial problems. I recovered from that operation and got on with my life.

"About 1979, I read about chelation therapy in one of the health magazines. This was a treatment described back then as a kind of 'chemical rotorooter' that cleaned out clogged arteries. Today I know that such a description isn't scientifically accurate but serves merely as an illustration for the lay reader. 'Wow!' I said to myself,

'This treatment sounds marvelous. I better tell my son about it.' So I telephoned my son John who was just then changing from a surgical residency in urology to begin the practice of general medicine in Humble, Texas. I read John exerpts from the chelation therapy magazine article.

"He listened and then said that the treatment commonly is employed for lead poisoning, but never had he heard of it being used for cleaning plaque out of hardened arteries.

"John told me, 'Forget it, Dad, it's just quackery. Don't you think if it was any good, I'd know about chelation therapy and be using it in my practice? Wouldn't I have read in the medical journals about such a marvelous way to reverse atherosclerosis? Well, the treatment isn't described in the journals for that purpose. So how could it be legitimate? I want you to stay away from those physicians who recommend chelation therapy, and don't bother yourself any further about such nonsense.' So I put it out of my mind," Jack Trowbridge said.

Dr. John Trowbridge Meets Chelation Therapy

A couple of years later, the light dawned for the younger Trowbridge. He read the first of several chelation therapy books written by Morton Walker, D.P.M. (*Chelation Therapy: How to Prevent or Reverse Hardening of the Arteries*, Stamford, Conn.: Freelance Communications, 1980). Moreover, while routinely using nutrition as treatment in his holistic medical practice, Dr. John Trowbridge heard other nutrition-oriented colleagues speak of remarkable recoveries from the administration of chelation therapy for degenerative diseases—especially for those conditions in which the underlying pathology is an interruption in blood flow. Together with a program of exercise, a prescribed regimen of highly concentrated nutrition (which frequently consists of megadoses of vitamins, minerals, and other food supplements) is an integral part of every patient's chelation procedure.

During Thanksgiving week, 1982, Dr. Trowbridge traveled to San Francisco to see his mother, who had undergone major surgery for seriously bleeding ulcers. Claire Trowbridge's surgery widened the passageway from her stomach into the duodenum, where an ulcer had caused damage and constriction of the stomach's pylorus. While he was in San Francisco, Dr. Trowbridge visited another physician-nutritionist, Robert Haskell, M.D., with whom he exchanged information on various treatment programs. Again, Dr. Trowbridge heard positive reports about chelation therapy.

Dr. Haskell told him, "Of all the regimens you can use to help your patients combat degenerative disease and restore their health, chelation therapy is the most powerful. It produces the greatest number of benefits to the body—far beyond those of improved blood flow. If you want to get your prescribed nutrition to those parts of the body in which they must work, John, chelation therapy is the way to do it."

Dr. Haskell amazed Dr. Trowbridge by showing him case histories of patients who showed marked improvements from chelation therapy. There was no denying the recovered patients' healthier laboratory test readings and clinical examination showings from having received their treatments. For example, Dr. Haskell showed him the case of Richard B. Davis, age 63, who before chelation therapy had high blood pressure, atherosclerosis, intermittent claudication (on and off leg cramps from poor circulation), angina (pain in the chest, sometimes radiating to the left arm, caused by a spasm of the coronary artery of the heart) that occurred both while the patient was active and at rest, and generalized arteriosclerosis.

Due to the severity of the angina, Mr. Davis could walk less than one block. Since he could not ascend a flight of stairs, he was forced to discontinue his work as an elevator repairman. His chest pain was unremitting.

"Our studies revealed elevated mercury and cadmium levels [both toxic metals] and severely elevated triglyceride levels [neutral fat in the blood which is a digestion product from dietary fat and sugars]. The patient was taking isoxsuprine [a vasodilator] four times daily and often needed nitroglycerine through the day and night to relieve his angina pains," Dr. Haskell explained. "The man's family history revealed that his mother and three brothers have heart disease; one brother has sustained a stroke; vascular disease is apparent in three brothers."

Dr. Haskell started Richard Davis on chelation therapy on March 30, 1982. After only five intravenous infusions with EDTA, Mr. Davis was able to walk three blocks and could also ascend stairs without feeling any angina pain. After 12 treatments, the patient needed to take isoxsuprine only three times per week. After receiving 30 chelation treatments his angina was completely gone.

By August of 1982, Davis had received 52 chelation treatments. His heavy metal poisoning from mercury and cadmium was gone. "The angina and intermittent claudication pains were completely gone [and have stayed away as of the present]. My patient can walk miles and miles. He climbs stairs with ease. He no longer takes isoxsuprine or nitroglycerine," said Dr. Haskell, "and his blood triglycerides have dropped from a high of 1,080 to a near-normal 223 milligrams percent. He feels a dramatic increase in energy, and his outlook on life has improved remarkably."

Dr. Trowbridge read through the medical records of numerous other patients being treated by Dr. Haskell. He interviewed some of them in person and listened to their amazing stories of feeling so much better after they took chelation treatments. He then decided to thoroughly investigate this dramatic new-but-old therapy.

First he read *The Chelation Answer* by Morton Walker, D.P.M. (New York: M. Evans, 1982). Then Dr. Trowbridge accumulated non-indexed medical journal articles on chelation therapy. These are clinical articles not available to the physician who merely requests "all the information on the subject" from his medical librarian. While non-indexed journals actually comprise about 90 percent of the world's scientific publications each year, medical libraries usually subscribe only to indexed journals.

Next, Dr. Trowbridge sought further information from the American College of Advancement in Medicine, the medical specialty organization that conducts research and keeps records on the results of the administration of chelation treatment. For the next eight months he intensively studied the materials and made personal observations by traveling to one chelation clinic after another. For instance, Dr. Trowbridge flew to Cottonwood, Alabama, and spent time with H. Ray Evers, M.D.; he then visited with Milan Packovich, M.D., in Washington (near Pittsburgh), Pennsylvania; Charles H. Farr, M.D., Ph.D. in Oklahoma City, Oklahoma, and a dozen others. Not one of these doctors reported negative results.

Every chelating physician that Dr. Trowbridge questioned was enthusiastic about the treatment. They opened their patient files to him. And the evidence was overwhelmingly affirmative that chelation therapy was effecting a medical revolution in overcoming degenerative diseases, just as 40 years before, antibiotic therapy effectively combatted infectious diseases. Dr. Trowbridge concluded that if medicine was worth practicing, it must include chelation therapy.

Jack and Claire Trowbridge Take Chelation Therapy

Dr. Trowbridge's cardiovascular disease patients as well as those who used him as their family doctor were introduced to chelation therapy in the early part of 1983. The doctor subsequently suggested to his parents that they come to Texas to receive chelation treatment.

Jack Trowbridge was absolutely ecstatic over the prospect, but he couldn't help teasing his son: "You mean it's not quackery? Not nonsense? Didn't you advise me to stay away from any doctor who suggested chelation treatment?"

Over a period of one year beginning in November 1983, Jack Trowbridge received 45 intravenous infusions of a synthetic amino acid, ethylene diamine tetraacetic acid (EDTA), for the purpose of chelation therapy.

"I now have good blood circulation," Jack said. Although his aortic aneurysm repair was reinforced by the treatment, the benefits from chelation therapy that this man has received go far beyond improvements in his blood flow.

"One of my problems was cold extremities," Jack added. "That's disappeared. I have warm feet again, no matter what the outside temperature is."

The spontaneously occurring burning and tingling sensations in two toes Jack had felt—like pins and needles—are now completely gone. These symptoms were indications of partial damage to peripheral nerves which now have been restored to normal functioning.

Trips in the Orient during his Air Force years had left Jack Trowbridge with a fungus infection of the toenails. Military doctors had spent 25 years trying to get rid of it without success. With the administration of chelation therapy alone, the toenails have improved. They've developed demarcation lines between new normal growth and the old fungus portions. "After my chelation therapy, the big toes have grown healthy nails that came in behind and shoved the diseased nails off," said the senior Trowbridge.

He no longer has arthritic joint complaints either. Jack wakes up these mornings feeling rested from a good night's sleep, and without the residual fatigue he used to have from tossing all night trying to find a comfortable position in bed. He is easily able to lift, pull, and push in doing odd jobs, renovations, minor construction work and general home repairs. Degenerative arthritis simply isn't a problem for him anymore.

"My once high blood pressure has come down and stabilized at 120/75, pretty good for being 70 years old," Jack Trowbridge said. "And besides all that, I just feel good."

Claire Trowbridge, who is 76, has also had excellent results from chelation therapy. She received 40 chelation treatments during the same period as her husband—from November 1983 to October 1984. Prior to chelation therapy, she tired easily as a result of having undergone a heart valve replacement for a faulty bicuspid aortic valve. Today, Claire has found new vitality. She is better able to handle stress, and has become a great source of strength to her family, whereas before, she never had the endurance.

"A year ago I told my husband that I was at the end of the trail. 'I don't think that I'm going to be here for long,' I said to Jack. 'Don't tell John, but all the symptoms I had before my heart surgery have returned. I am losing my balance again; to walk, I must hold onto the furniture or the walls; my heart muscle is hurting; my arms feel heavy; I'm having difficulty breathing; I feel stress from every situation; I'm just not well. I certainly don't want to go through any more heart valve surgery. It's ridiculous! I can't keep changing heart valves to stay alive. I figure the Good Lord is calling me.' "

Jack Trowbridge would have done anything to help his wife, but he was at a loss as to how to proceed.

"My cardiologist put me on hypertension pills because my blood pressure was too high," continued Claire. "But even with the medicine my blood pressure either stayed up or it yoyoed up and down.

"I also started to forget words. I could be talking about something as simple as water; I'd get to the word 'water' and not be able to recall the word to say. I couldn't think," Claire explained.

"A painful Morton's neuroma in the fourth toe of my left foot was unsuccessfully operated on in 1981. I limped all the time. But since I have taken chelation therapy, I don't limp anymore. The pain is gone.

"Jack and John arranged for me to travel to Houston for the chelation treatments. After receiving the fifth IV [intravenous] injection, I couldn't believe what was happening to me," Mrs. Trowbridge continued. "I said to Jack, 'This is a miracle; I never felt better in my life.' The more IVs I took, the better I felt.

"My balance has completely returned; I can look up and down without getting dizzy. My breathing got easier. My heart muscles stopped hurting. My blood pressure is normal, too. All of my uncomfortable symptoms are gone. It's as if I've come back from nearly being dead, and all because of the chelation therapy my son has given to me. I'm so proud of what John is doing for people."

Intravenous (IV) Chelation Therapy

Hardening of the arteries is a growing threat to every American. We are currently facing a very real epidemic of this illness—with symptoms ranging from poor circulation in the extremities to kidney disorders and heart disease. It is estimated that 67.7 percent of all the disease-precipitated deaths in this country (heart attack 54.7 percent, stroke 13 percent) are the result of one form or another of hardening of the arteries.

A person diagnosed as having atherosclerosis is usually offered very few choices in dealing with the illness. If the blocked arteries are large enough to be operated upon, the victim takes his chances with bypass or "cleanout" surgery. But, if the stricken blood vessels are too small for surgical techniques, then the patient must become resigned to living with this seemingly incurable and progressive disease.

Unbeknownst to most people, however, there is a unique medical process that can clean out the arteries and renew blood flow throughout the entire body—without surgery! This exciting process is intravenous chelation therapy. Certain nutrient, or chemical, agents used for the chelation process include vitamin C, lactated Ringer's solution (which resembles the blood serum in its salt constituents), EDTA (ethylene diamine tetraacetic acid), some other weak organic acids, plus other agents. By far, the most frequently used agent in chelation therapy is EDTA.

As mentioned previously, EDTA chelation therapy consists of intravenous infusions of a synthesized amino acid, a protein-like substance made in the laboratory. Scientists have demonstrated that when the EDTA solution is injected into the bloodstream, just one of the beneficial things it does is trigger the breakdown of components of plaque and lock onto, or chelate, heavy metals. Plaque is the internal "corrosion" that commonly clogs the arteries of middle-aged and elderly (and some young) people. EDTA' stimulates the processes by which the cellular components of the plaque, such as heavy metals, mucopolysaccharides, calcium, cholesterol, collagen, fibrin, foreign proteins, and other debris release their hold on the internal wall of the arteries. These particles then become a part of the EDTA molecular solution and leave the bloodstream through the kidneys to be finally eliminated in the urine. As this occurs, the hardened arteries become more flexible. The narrowing of their central channel (the lumen) is halted, and the blood flow is unclogged.

Moreover, tests reveal another benefit from chelation therapy. EDTA IV injections can help pull calcium from other parts of the body in which it is abnormally deposited, such as in traumatized tendons, inflamed bursae, kidney stones, arthritic joints, and strained ligaments. But IV EDTA does *not* remove calcium from the bones and teeth, where the mineral serves a very useful purpose. Rather, EDTA chelation therapy tends to strengthen the bone by reactivating dormant but healthy bone-forming cells. For this reason, IV EDTA and its associated nutritional oral chelating agents have been useful in treating osteoporosis.

Thermograms, plethysmograms, the doppler ultrasound, and other diagnostic tests taken before and after chelation treatment reveal that impaired circulation is often restored to normal by this medical process. After the clogging material is removed from the human arterial wall, a smooth, clean, and nearly unblocked surface is thought to be left behind.

Experiments Prove that Chelation Therapy Unclogs Arteries

The smoothing of the arterial wall and the removal of calcium have been well demonstrated in autopsied laboratory animals that received chelation treatment.

Interestingly, however, even before animal experiments proved the efficacy of intravenous EDTA, it was used on human subjects for its therapeutic effect. The earliest reported research using EDTA for removal of plaque-producing calcium deposits was conducted in 1946 at the University of Zurich, and in 1947 and 1948 at the University of Bern.

A paper, "New Treatment of Corneal Opacities," written by W. Grant, M.D. (*Archives of Ophthalmology*, volume 48, 1952, pp. 6-81) described the use of EDTA chelation therapy as a solution for removing calcium from the eyes of human patients with post-keratitis corneal opacities which had resulted in cataracts.

In the laboratory, Drs. L. E. Bolick and D. H. Blankenhorn demonstrated the effectiveness of EDTA for the removal of calcium from atheromatous arterial plaques from dissected arteries. Total calcium content of coronary vessels and the rate of calcium removal were determined.

Bolick and Blankenhorn's article, "A Quantitative Study of Coronary Artery Calcification," (*American Journal of Pathology*, volume 39, 1961, pp. 511-517), indicated that coronary artery atheromatous calcifications can be as extensive as aortic lesions and that in both locations the plaques occur in two different forms. One form contained calcium, which, when removed, left behind hematoxylin-ringed lacunae. Hematoxylin is a chemical dye that takes on the color qualities of the tissue on which it is being used ás a stain. Lacunae are small cavities, or depressions. Thus, colored rings of depression remained in the arteries when the calcium was slowly extracted by EDTA. The other form of calcification showed no lacunae and appeared to be more diffusely dispersed. The calcium content of this second type of plaque was more rapidly extracted by EDTA.

An article published in 1963 in the *Journal of Chronic Diseases*, volume 16, pp. 329-333, entitled "Some *in Vitro* Effects of Chelation-II Animal Experimentation," by Drs. A. Koen, D.S. McCann, and A. J. Boyle, described the results of subcutaneous injections of magnesium disodium EDTA on rabbits. The animals had been fed with a cholesterol-enriched diet. The researchers found that following the EDTA injections, the surface of the rabbits' aortae showed diminished formation of atheromatous plaques and a marked decrease in phospholipids. They concluded that chelation therapy resulted in slower synthesis and more rapid destruction of phospholipids, as well as an increased turnover of phospate. Phosphates and phospholipids are important factors in the clogging of human arteries.

That EDTA is able to remove calcium from the arterial wall was conclusively shown in a study by Fred Walker, Ph.D. and outlined in his doctoral thesis, "The Effects of EDTA Chelation Therapy on Plaque, Calcium, and Mineral Metabolism in Arteriosclerotic Rabbits." (Available at the University Microfilm International Library in Ann Arbor, Michigan 48016.) Walker fed New Zealand albino rabbits an atherogenic diet for 23 weeks, which produced in them calcified aortic plaques with marked elevation of serum cholesterol levels to approximately 1,200 mg/dL.

One month after they were taken off this artery-clogging diet, the rabbits were treated on alternating days with disodium EDTA (50 mg/kg body weight) by IV injection into the marginal ear vein. Each animal received 20 infusions. Six weeks after completion of EDTA chelation therapy, the animals were sacrificed and their aortae examined for tissue calcium—both quantitatively by direct micro-complexometric analysis, and histologically.

The rabbits given EDTA exhibited significantly less ($P=.05$) aortic calcium. (A "p-value" at this low level means the results are highly unlikely to be a matter of "chance" in this experiment.) The EDTA treated rabbits showed 300 mcg/gm of tissue, when compared with those animals treated with normal salt solution (saline), which showed 635 mcg/mg of tissue. Furthermore, the animals that received no infusions showed an even greater aortic calcium content of 778 mcg/mg of tissue.

Obvious calcified plaques could be seen in non-infused animals while none were noted in those which had received EDTA. These results indicated conclusively that disodium EDTA chelation therapy can cause the removal of plaque calcium from the aortae of athero-sclerotic rabbits, contributing to a reduction in both size and number of atheromatous lesions.

The EDTA Chelation Therapy Program

IV chelation therapy has significantly helped over 500,000 Americans, most of them victims of hardening of the arteries. The American College of Advancement in Medicine (ACAM), the medical organization whose members specialize in giving this treatment, documents numerous health benefits from chelation therapy. For example, high blood pressure goes down and usually becomes normal; hands and feet grow warmer with improved blood flow; impending kidney problems are averted; the chances of stroke and heart attack are greatly reduced or eliminated; pain caused by cancer is lessened and cancer cells are more able to be exposed to the body's natural immune processes; symptoms of such degenerative diseases as lupus erythematosis, Parkinson's disease, multiple sclerosis, amyotrophic lateral sclerosis (Lou Gehrig's disease), senile dementia, Alzheimer's disease, cataracts, glaucoma, macular degeneration in the eye, diabetes, diabetic retinopathy, intermittent claudication, impotency, angina, arthritis, arteriosclerosis, osteoporosis, radiation toxicity, cirrhosis, schizophrenia, gangrene, varicose veins, hypercalcemia, Raynaud's disease, scleroderma, digitalis intoxication, heavy metal poisoning, sickle cell anemia, high serum cholesterol, and many more conditions where the underlying pathology appears to be an interruption in blood flow or an elevated incidence of free radical pathology, are reduced or eliminated altogether.

During and after treatment, IV EDTA patients are encouraged by the supervising chelating physician to change to a healthier lifestyle. They are given programs of daily exercise, a natural way to self-chelation, as the weak organic chelator, lactic acid, is a byproduct of muscular activity. Also prescribed for patients are high doses of oral chelating and assisting agents in the form of vitamins, minerals, amino acids, protomorphogens, enzymes, and other nutrients, all designed to help the arteries stay healthy and flexible. Additionally, patients are advised to have periodic hair mineral analyses to determine precisely what mineral supplements they should take to maintain the body's natural chemistry.

The IV infusion of EDTA, however, is the key to restoring victims of degenerative diseases to improved health and vitality—relatively quickly. Sometimes as few as 15 or 20 treatments with EDTA are administered.

Usually, however, a series of 24, 36, or more injections are given over several months. The patient receives each "IV drip" for from three to five hours once or twice (occasionally three times) a week. The number of injections, their frequency, and the speed of the infusions depend on the extent of a patient's medical problems. Based on diagnostic guidelines, the chelating physician may be able to predict the number of IV treatments required by the patient. (To check physician training and chelation therapy certification contact the American College of Advancement in Medicine, 23121 Verdugo Drive, Suite 204, Laguna Hills, California 92653; (800) 532-3688 (outside California); (714) 583-7666 (in California).

Creation of the intravenous chelation solution follows a specific protocol recommended by the ACAM, with variations made by individual chelating physicians. One such solutions, formulated by Dr. Trowbridge, follows the ACAM protocol. This formulation may be typical of ingredients and their dosages made up by other chelating physicians. A patient should be aware of the solution he is receiving.

The constant solution outlined below usually will not change unless by order of the physician or because of a patient's anticipated allergic reaction to one of the ingredients in Dr. Trowbridge's basic formula for a chelation solution prepared in 500 ml of sterile water for intravenous infusion.

Draw up the listed ingredients in a 50-ml syringe, freshly opened for each preparation session. Before drawing up, use a syringe to remove about 30 ml of the carrier solution (sterile water) from the IV bottle.

Name of Constituent	Concentration in mg/ml	X x	Amount ml	= Total = mg
Magnesium chloride - $MgCl_2$	200 mg/ml	9 ml	1,800 mg	
Hydrochloric acid - HCl	2 mg/ml	6 ml	12 mg	
Potassium chloride - KCl	40 mEq/ml	3 ml	120 mEq	
Thiamine (vitamin B-1)	100 mg/ml	3 ml	300 mg	
Niacinamide (vitamin B-3)	100 mg/ml	3 ml	300 mg	
Pyridoxine (vitamin B-6)	100 mg/ml	3 ml	300 mg	
Dexpanthenol (vitamin B-5)	250 mg/ml	3 ml	750 mg	
Sodium Thiosalicylate - Thyodyne (Pharm-A-Sist[R])	50 mg/ml	3 ml	150 mg	
Cyanocobalamin (vitamin B-12)	1000 mg/ml	1 ml	1,000 mcg	
Ascorbic Acid (vitamin C)	500 mg/ml	50 ml	25,000 mg	

The ascorbic acid content usually will not change, unless by physician order. Draw up the ascorbic acid in the 50-ml syringe just used for making the constant solution.

The following additions or variable solution parts should only be utilized by direct and clear physician order. These constituents will be added, depending on the individual patient's health need.

The following ingredients may be drawn into a 30-ml syringe or into the 50-ml syringe which has already been used for making the constant solution:

Lidocaine	20 mg/ml	6 ml	120 mg
(Possibly omit lidocaine altogether)			
Niacinamide (vitamin B-3)	100 mg/ml	3-6 ml	300-600 mg

Usually this extra niacinamide is added only for the treatment of peripheral vascular disease and only at or after the fourth IV.

Heparin	5,000 units	1 ml	5,000 units

Never give heparin if the patient is taking anticoagulant medication. (Possibly omit this addition.)

Methionine 100 mg/ml; Inositol 100 mg/ml; choline 100 mg/ml; note that 6 ml=600 mg each; administered every sixth treatment, unless the physician orders "no MIC."

EDTA	150 mg/ml	0-20 =	0-3.0 g

EDTA dosage varies according to patient's clinical condition and laboratory testing results.

Oral chelation therapy works much slower than the intravenous method, and by a somewhat different process, but both can eventually bring about beneficial effects for the body and the mind. If you can't wait for oral chelation therapy to work alone, because of the presence of distressing disease symptoms and signs, then IV chelation therapy is probably the preferred treatment. An oral chelating program, prescribed under a holistic physician's supervision, makes sense before, during, and after IV EDTA therapy.

Thanks to both types of chelation therapy, people with hardening of the arteries and/or free radical pathology can hope to reverse symptoms.

But what about the millions of patients suffering with various forms of degenerative disease who don't know about EDTA chelation therapy? Who fail even to get the oral chelating advantages of vitamins, minerals, protomorphogens, enzymes, amino acids, antioxidants, and other supplemental nutrients? Many sufferers are also denied the option of surgery, for a variety of reasons: lack of funds, no health insurance, just plain ignorance about health matters, an unhealthy lifestyle, a disinterested family doctor, misinformation about the treatment from competing physicians.

Arterial surgery is restricted to the larger blood vessels. Hardening of the arteries affects the circulatory system of the entire body. Arterial clogging takes place in the brain, causing senility and stroke; in the cardiac region, affecting heart and lungs; in the abdominal region, which impairs blood flow to the kidneys, liver, pancreas and other organs; in the common iliac arteries, reducing blood flow to the genitals and legs; and in the small popliteal vessels around the knees, which eventually causes gangrene of the feet. In these cases, chelation therapy is especially valuable, because injections of the EDTA solution can reach and affect even the smallest capillaries which, under normal circumstances, are inoperable.

Is Chelation Therapy Accepted by Organized Medicine?

For all the remarkable benefits and usefulness of intravenous chelation therapy, it seems incredible that it is not commonly used or even considered by the medical community at large as a cure (or even part of the care) for atherosclerosis. Although it has been used therapeutically in the United States for lead poisoning and other heavy metal toxicities since 1948, and for hardening of the arteries since 1952, chelation therapy is fraught with controversy among physicians. Some are vehemently against the treatment; others have totally integrated it into their practices.

There are, indeed, proponents who swear by intravenous chelation therapy. These doctors take it themselves, and give it to their loved ones and their patients. Such doctors refuse to follow organized medicine's official dogmatic policy and, instead, courageously accept the harassment of medical colleagues who relentlessly oppose the administration of the EDTA infusion against atherosclerosis. Unquestionably, chelating physicians are 20th-century Semmelweisses.

Ignaz P. Semmelweiss (1818-1865) was ridiculed by fellow physicians and hounded into insanity and eventually death. Why? Because he wanted his colleagues to wash their hands after assisting in the birth of one baby and before going on to the next. In 1845, Semmelweiss was the first to recognize the connection of infectious puerperal septicemia to childbed fever, an infection of the uterus following childbirth. When obstetricians finally started washing their hands, deaths from childbed fever among newly delivered mothers were markedly reduced. The position of chelating physicians today is comparable to that of Semmelweiss in his day.

Though EDTA chelation therapy is equally effective as a treatment for hardening of the arteries as it is for heavy metal poisoning, it is still widely opposed by "medical mainstream" practitioners and especially by most cardiovascular and peripheral vascular surgeons. One reason they resist chelation therapy is that they seem not to have done their homework. Apparently they are unaware of the extensive clinical research which has been carried out by users of the therapy, mainly by those chelating physician-members of the ACAM.

More than 1,800 medical journal articles have positively evaluated EDTA chelation therapy, about 60 of which were published within the past five years. However, because, by and large, medical traditionalists control editorial policy of standard medical journals, the papers on current clinical studies had to be published in non-indexed, non-supervised journals. Editorial boards subject to the stranglehold of establishment medicine refuse to publish anything about the clinical documentation relating to the efficacy of chelation therapy. Articles on controlled clinical chelation studies are mostly printed in *The Journal of Holistic Medicine*, the *Townsend Letter for Doctors*, the *Journal of Advancement in Medicine, Health Consciousness*, and others. The conservative adherents of American organized medicine apparently never read these journals. Consequently, they still spout the old inaccuracies, erroneous statements offered to explain chelation therapy benefits in publications from prior years, such as 1954 or 1963.

As we said earlier, the chelation treatment has been shown to heal a variety of malfunctions and disabilities where the underlying pathology is an interference in the individual's blood flow and damage from free radical pathology. (Free radical pathology will be discussed at length in the sections to follow.) Healing is accomplished with great safety. Flushing the arteries with intravenous infusions of EDTA or some other intravenous chelating agent can bring fresh blood and oxygen to the tissues and can aid in the healing process. When this procedure is performed properly, by following the protocol published by the American College of Advancement in Medicine, it is an extremely scientific and highly effective system of circulatory treatment.

Health care consumers should know about IV chelation therapy as an alternative to coronary artery bypass and other forms of heart and blood vessel surgery. As it now stands, someone suffering from hardening of the arteries generally receives *incomplete* information or *no* information at all about alternatives to toxic drugs or dangerous surgery, which poses serious questions about the meaning of "informed consent" and whether medical malpractice is being committed. Chelation therapy is rarely offered, perhaps because the patient's family doctor or the medical specialist to whom he or she has been referred possesses insufficient knowledge about the procedure.

How Safe is IV Chelation Therapy?

Intravenous chelation therapy is safe, proved to be more than three times as safe as taking an aspirin, according to the biotoxicological tests performed on laboratory animals. The "LD-50" of EDTA is calculated at 2000 milligrams (mg) per kilogram (kg) of body weight of a human being, while aspirin has an "LD-50" of only 558 mg per kg. (LD-50 stands for the "lethal dose 50" or the dose of a substance which is fatal to 50 percent of the test subjects it is administered to.) In a test group of one-kilogram animals, 558 mg of aspirin would probably kill half of them. But it would take 2000 mg of EDTA to kill the same number.

Since 1954, when two patients developed kidney complications and died, no deaths have resulted directly and solely from the use of chelation therapy. But this tragedy was caused by the inadvertant administration of an excessive dosage of IV EDTA—10 grams every day, five days a week, for three weeks. Today, it is known that no more, and frequently less, than three grams of the chelating agent on an average of only twice a week should be given. Also, thirty years ago, the intravenous infusion was allowed to drip into the patient's vein exceedingly fast—too fast. Today, three to five hours must be taken for the slow drip to filter into the bloodstream.

Yet, doctors who practice orthodox medicine and who oppose the use of chelation therapy still cite those deaths as an indication that chelation therapy is unsafe. It goes without saying that no physician specializing in chelation therapy who follows the ACAM protocol today would administer the treatment in the obviously risky way it was given to patients before 1954.

Nor is chelation therapy responsible for kidney damage, when the physician follows the ACAM protocol. By monitoring a patient's kidneys with 24-hour creatinine clearance measurements and blood urea nitrogen (BUN) tests the doctor assures the patient's safety. Such tests also have shown that malfunctioning kidneys often become "almost like new," according to the published research of chelating physicians Edward W. McDonagh, D.O., Charles J. Rudolph, D.O., Ph.D., and Emanuel Cheraskin, M.D., D.M.D., all of Gladstone, Missouri.

The few adverse side effects that could develop are minor compared to the advantages of chelation therapy.

The risk-benefit ratio is overwhelmingly on the side of benefits.

One occasional side effect is a drop in blood pressure, which helps the patient with hypertension. Another possible side effect is hypoglycemia; but a drop in blood sugar is easily counteracted if the patient eats during the IV drip. The doctor is ever watchful for signs of hypocalcemia and keeps handy a syringe of calcium solution for intravenous injection in case it's needed. Other incidental side effects might include dizziness, nausea, tingling of the skin around the mouth, and burning at the site of injection. Patients urinate much more frequently during the infusion.

Chelating physicians believe that only by reversing such diseases as atherosclerosis, or by preventing them altogether, will a person be able to live out his allotted life span. Many prominent scientists claim that human beings are genetically programmed to live a *healthy* 120 years. People who live in industrialized Western countries, unfortunately, survive to little more than half that age, due, in many cases, to the debilitating and fatal effects of hardening of the arteries.

The Man Who Thwarted Predictable Death

Death at about one half his life expectancy was the predictable fate of Edward I. Spannoza, a Brooklyn, New York, resident who finally sought help from chelating physician Warren M. Levin, M.D., of New York City. Mr. Spannoza was 65 years old at the time of his first consultation with Dr. Levin, in August 1977. In January 1976 he was hospitalized for three weeks for a "mild" sub-endocardial (heart muscle) infarct. Such an infarct is an area of heart tissue that has been deprived of its blood supply because of a clot within the artery. This condition can cause sudden death in 50 percent of those it strikes; the rest suffer slow death through degeneration.

"As far back as I can remember," said Spannoza, "I've had high blood pressure, for which I never received any medication. But after my heart attack, I went on heart medicines like Inderal™ and Isordil™ and Valium™. At other times the cardiologist prescribed other heart medicines such as quinidine and Hydrodiuril™ -Apresoline™."

But even with the medication the man's blood pressure stayed high—150/100 sitting and 160/105 standing. He suffered mostly from angina, chronic fatigue, constant weakness, and irregular heartbeat. He also had insomnia, diminished libido, impotence, backaches, impaired memory, and painful arthritis of the hip.

"At his initial physical examination and laboratory workup," reports Dr. Levin, "my patient demonstrated abnormalities on his electrocardiogram, hypothyroidism, borderline serum magnesium, elevated levels of lead and cadmium in his hair mineral analysis, and a creatinine clearance of 44, which indicated a significant impairment of blood flow through the kidneys. He also demonstrated a low serum T-4, a slightly elevated TSH, and a slow Achilles tendon reflex, all of which confirm the suspected presence of hypothyroidism.

"More than that, the patient also showed significant undigested starch in his stool. Glucose tolerance testing indicated that he had a latent diabetes with a reactive hypoglycemia. Non-invasive studies of the circulation showed diminished pulses in the toes. A provocative lead test with calcium EDTA [Versenate™] produced a 24-hour lead excretion of well over 300 micrograms per day." Mr. Spannoza was a victim of lead poisoning.

Dr. Levin started Spannoza on a course of chelation therapy, which would include annual booster injections. "As of August 1984 the patient, at age 72, is taking no cardiac or antihypertensive medications," said Dr. Levin. "He has no arrhythmia; his energy is excellent. His libido has returned and he is no longer impotent. The pulses to his toes are now excellent; the creatinine clearance is above average for his age, indicating a dramatic improvement in blood flow through the kidneys; his electrocardiogram, although still abnormal, shows significant improvement. He takes no medication, his blood pressure is completely normal, and his most recent lead excretion test is normal."

Ed Spannoza reports that, since the end of his first series of 36 chelation treatments, six years ago, his backaches have gone, and that he is no longer bothered by pain in his hip from degenerative arthritis. His memory has improved so much that he's come out of retirement to assist his grandson in a new business venture.

Dr. Levin incidentally commented on the health insurance industry's attitude toward chelation therapy as a viable and acceptable procedure. Dr. Levin wrote: "Lead and cadmium toxicity are known to be capable of causing hypertension. Hypothyroidism aggravates hypertension and the tendency to coronary artery disease. Yet, when this patient [Spannoza] asked his health insurance company about coverage he was denied payment because his treatment was not 'usual and customary,' while all of the ineffective treatment that he had been receiving, including the diuretics which aggravated his arrhythmia and fatigue, were paid for without question! What a condemnation of the usual and customary medical treatment in this country!"

Free Radical Pathology

New discoveries about free radical pathology are providing medical scientists with a cogent explanation of why and how high dosage nutrition in the form of oral chelating agents and intravenous chelation therapy work to bring dysfunctioning body and brain cells back to good repair. We have frequently alluded to the free radical concept of disease. People have been exhibiting signs and symptoms of deterioration from a source of pathology heretofore unexplained. This section will explain that source—known as "free radical pathology."

"Free Radical Pathology in Age-Associated Diseases: Treatment with EDTA Chelation, Nutrition and Antioxidants," (*Journal of Holistic Medicine*, volume 6, number 1, Spring/Summer 1984) by Elmer M. Cranton, M.D., of Trout Dale, Virginia, a past vice president of the ACAM and past president of the American Holistic Medical Association, and James P. Frackelton, MD., of Cleveland, Ohio, past president of the ACAM and vice-chairman of the American Board of Chelation Therapy, states "...[The free radical concept of disease] is as revolutionary and profound in its implication for medicine as was the germ theory and science of microbiology which made possible development of effective treatments for infectious diseases. The free radical concept explains contradictory epidemiologic and clinical observations and provides a scientific basis for treatment and prevention of the major causes of disability and death—atherosclerosis, dementia, cancer, arthritis, and other age-related diseases."

The two chelating physicians go on to explain that free radicals are indiscriminately reactive molecules and molecular fragments that interact aggressively with other molecules in your body to rapidly create new unbalanced atoms. A free radical has an unpaired electron in an outer atomic orbit, causing it to be highly unstable and to react almost instantaneously with any substance in its vicinity. This reaction often tosses free radicals in all directions and damages the cells. Such harm begins as a result of exposure to X-rays, gamma rays, cosmic radiation, ultraviolet light from the sun, cigarette smoke, automobile exhaust fumes, food additives, toxic metals in drinking water, and other ecological phenomena to which each of us is continuously exposed in our highly technological environment.

Free radicals are harmful to the body because when photons of radiation knock electrons out of orbiting atomic rings, the free radicals penetrate living tissues, causing peroxidation of unsaturated fatty acids in cell membranes. Highly reactive free radical molecules include hydroxyl radicals, superoxide radicals, and excited or singlet state oxygen that produce hydrogen peroxide and fat peroxides which cause cell damage.

To prevent uncontrolled multiplication of free radicals, which would eventually kill all the cells in the body, human cells utilize more than a dozen antioxidant control systems. Such control mechanisms involve several enzymes, including catalase, superoxide dismutase (SOD), glutathione peroxidase, and others, in conjunction with vitamins C, E, A (beta carotene), the trace element selenium, and other food substances. Insufficient quantities of the various necessary food substances in your diet will result in too few antioxidants to stop the free radical pathology that you cannot escape being exposed to.

When functioning properly, your antioxidant systems suppress reactions from excessive free radicals so healthful biological processes can go on without undesirable cellular and molecular damage. Otherwise, free radicals will multiply rapidly, much like a nuclear chain reaction, disrupting cell membranes, damaging enzymatic proteins, interfering with both active and passive transport of nutrients across cell membranes. Mutagenic damage is bound to take place, which invariably leads to cancer.

Specific molecular food substances tend to prevent the formation of abnormally functioning or malignant cells. Others are a factor in the production of free radical control enzymes absolutely necessary to help you cope with the myriad antigens, carcinogens, atherogens, pathogens, allergens, and other disease-producing elements that you are subjected to every day. The chemical industry admits that over 60,000 man-made pollutants have been added to our environment. Plus, Federal estimates suggest that we are exposed to 5,000 substances intentionally added to our foods and to some 10,000 more that are unintentionally included as a result of production or packaging. Indeed, probably 10,000 pollutants attack your body processes every day. More than mutagenesis, free-radical-controlled enzymes prevent, or act therapeutically against, almost all the degenerative diseases.

The food substances in the intravenous infusion solution and in the oral chelating agents prescribed by your chelating physician give rise to the free-radical-controlling enzymes such as superoxide dismutase (SOD). And the amount of SOD you possess is in direct proportion to your life span and life expectancy. SOD usually is the fifth most prevalent protein molecule in the human body, and the more you have the longer your life expectancy.

Human beings possess the highest concentration of SOD, which allows them to live up to the potential of their genetic codes, which, we have mentioned, is 120 years. People who live in industrialized countries invariably have shortened life expectancies, probably because they use up SOD too fast, as the result of an abusive lifestyle and their unending exposure to technological pollutants. It may also be that the number of non-enzymatic free radical scavengers, some of which are consumed quickly on a one-to-one ratio when neutralizing free radicals, are expended inordinately fast. The non-enzymatic free radical scavengers include cholesterol, glutathione, cysteine, methionine, tyrosine, pro-vitamin A, vitamin E, vitamin C, glucocorticosteroids, and selenium.

According to Drs. Frackelton and Cranton, "Enzymes involved in free radical protection require trace elements or B vitamins as co-enzymes. The trace elements copper, zinc, and manganese are essential to the superoxide dismutases; selenium is essential to glutathione peroxidase; and iron is necessary for catalase and other forms of peroxidase. Adequate dietary intake of these trace elements is necessary for protection against free radical produced disease." Two sure ways to get adequate dietary intake of trace elements, co-enzymes, non-enzymatic free radical scavengers and other nutrient elements that work against free radicals is in IV chelation therapy and in oral chelation agents.

Chelation is scientifically defined as a chemical reaction between a metal ion and a complexing agent, which results in the formation of a stable ring structure incorporating the metal ion. The complexing, or chelating, agent (often amino acid proteins) controls metal ions by blocking their reactive sites and preventing them from causing any possible adverse reactions, for example, free radical pathology. Minerals, especially, are vulnerable to many undesirable reactions before they are properly absorbed by human and animal bodies.

Chelation goes on continually inside the human body. For instance, hemoglobin, the red part of blood, is a chelate of iron. The ability of a mineral that you have eaten to undergo chelation in your own body depends on environment. It is affected by ecological changes. All the physical, chemical, and biological properties of your system determine if, whether, and how much, complexing will occur.

Literally thousands of chelations are taking place in your body every minute, particularly if you are in a stressful situation, a polluted area, or any other harmful environment.

Tobacco smoke in particular contains elements destructive to the enzymes. Polynuclear aromatic hydrocarbons found in tobacco tar and tobacco combustion produce a variety of free radicals, including singlet oxygen, the most common destructive agent. The only known protection against singlet oxygen is taking beta carotene, or pro-vitamin A, the yellow pigment found in carrots and other vegetables and fruit. Recent epidemiologic evidence shows that increased intake of vitamin A reduces incidence of cancer, even in smokers.

How Chelation Therapy Improves Oxygenation

IV chelation treatment is considered one of the nutritional therapies. It helps vitamins, fats, hormones, enzymes, proteins, minerals, raw glandular extracts, carbohydrates, and other food substances to complete their metabolic actions in the body. Such nutrients help the body to detoxify itself.

When you ingest such poisonous substances as heavy metals in drinking water, sulfites as vegetable preservatives, growth hormones in beef, antibiotics in pork, or nitrites in luncheon meats, the EDTA chelating agent works to detoxify the poison by molecular action. It increases the amount of oxygen used by the cellular tissue.

There are approximately 75 trillion cells in the human body, and each of these cells needs oxygen (among other elements) to function. When you receive intravenous chelation therapy—or even ingest oral chelating agents—you are helping all the cells utilize their oxygen. Nutritional scientists who administer the treatments do not know exactly how IV and oral chelators work. Only a few reactions are known relative to the vast numbers that exist, and the scientists are still studying them.

What is known is that since every body cell needs oxygen to function, by assisting in the oxygenation process, IV EDTA and oral chelating agents can, and do, significantly affect health and health-related problems, especially those involving the nerves, sex organs, and the cardiovascular system.

The body sometimes suffers from an oxygen drag. People frequently don't breathe deeply enough or they live in a polluted atmosphere. For example, cigarette smokers and toll-takers at bridges, tunnels, and on superhighways suffer from oxygen depletion because they constantly breathe in the carbon monoxide in cigarette smoke and automobile exhaust fumes. These people often develop degenerative diseases, such as heart disease, diabetes, and cancer, the three most common causes of death in the United States. Such victims desperately need to take EDTA chelation therapy and, under the supervision of a doctor trained in nutrition therapy, should continue to take oral chelating agents throughout their working lives. Such patients probably have insufficient oxygen to eliminate these health problems on their own.

Chelation therapy, both intravenous and oral, helps to prevent or overcome six of the 10 big killer diseases of Americans, which are, in order of frequency, heart disease, cancer, diabetes, stroke, accidents, pneumonia, cirrhosis of the liver, arteriosclerosis, suicides, and infant death. All except infant death, suicide, pneumonia and accidents are prevented or reversed by the use of chelation therapy.

There are strong indications that IV chelation therapy accompanied by prescribed oral chelating agents has a positive effect on very active people such as athletes, outdoor laborers, and others engaged in physically demanding jobs. Professional and amateur athletes who take orally-chelating type food supplements report that they have markedly increased stamina. This in itself suggests that chelation therapy provides the tissues with an abundant supply of oxygen. Imagine how much more stamina an athlete would have if he took IV chelation therapy on a preventive basis.

Sexual Help From Chelation Therapy

Chelation therapy has a profound effect on sexual performance. Many physicians who treat sexual dysfunction with nutrition consider IV EDTA, along with the oral chelating agents, as "love nutrients," because without them, the love lives of many of their patients would not exist. Chelation therapy can improve your sexual energy—people lacking stamina usually don't want anything to do with sex. There shouldn't be any sexual burnout for someone who, on a regular preventive basis takes intravenous EDTA and takes doctor-prescribed orally-chelating nutrients.

Middle-aged and older women can use the love nutrients in chelation therapy to recapture the sexual joys of youth. Many men who have been sexually inactive find that after treatment with EDTA injections and capsules, drops, powders, tablets, or other forms of nutrition therapy can engage in frequent love sessions. Blockage of blood flow to the genitals is eliminated.

Benson Morrison, age 75, of Port Arthur, Texas, who retired from an oil company 10 years ago after performing hard physical work all of his life, received chelation therapy under the medical supervision of Dr. Trowbridge, for the specific purpose of unclogging the carotid arteries in his neck. A blockage of blood to the brain had been causing Morrison bouts of dizziness and fainting. He was also concerned about long-standing impotence.

"My sex life had just died! During the last seven years, everything just went caflooey—no erection anymore," said Morrison. "But these [chelation] treatments have done me good.

"The way it started, I had a bad cold. He [Dr. Trowbridge] loaded me with a bunch of vitamin pills—they seemed to do good. Then we talked about taking a few of these treatments to see how they would affect my head. I said, 'OK, I'll do that,' and I did.

"Now I'm thrilled about the situation. I decided that if it [chelation therapy] would work on my head, why, it would work on the rest of the arteries. I noticed that at about the sixth treatment everything was coming back to me. I got erections again." Benson Morrison provided us with signed releases permitting us to tell his story so that others of the 10 million American men with erectile difficulties might find a possible solution to their impotence.

Morrison added that he was experiencing other benefits from chelation therapy, including elimination of his feelings of faintness. He said: "I couldn't walk too far before, maybe just a little way, and then I'd feel like I was going to black out. The same thing happened after driving my car. Then that all stopped [from the chelation treatment]. And I can breathe better—real deep and it doesn't hurt."

Chelation Therapy for Arthritis Symptoms

Veterinarian Lloyd S. McKibbin of Wheatley, Ontario, Canada, who treats arthritic thoroughbred race horses with chelation therapy, heard the pathetic complaints of his friend Grant Bowman, a 46-year-old manager of a feed mill, also in rural Wheatley. Bowman had been an athlete all his life, mostly playing baseball and hockey. But sports could no longer be part of his activities because he suffered severely from osteoarthritis.

From 1977 to 1981, the pain and swelling of Bowman's knees, ankles, wrists, fingers, and back had become so serious that not only was he forced to quit all athletics but he could barely perform his job, which required lifting 40- and 80- pound bags of animal feed. Since he lived only 100 yards from his place of work, he considered getting a golf cart to travel to the mill because the short walk had become such a painful chore. A rheumatologist who diagnosed Bowman's osteoarthritis prescribed Indocin™ for him. The drug provided some temporary relief from his pain but it also caused him much stomach distress.

At that point Dr. McKibbin referred his friend to Richard E. Tapert, D.O., Medical Director of the Family Health Clinic in Detroit, Michigan. Bowman made his first visit to this chelating physician in June 1981. After conducting his own clinical and laboratory tests and confirming the patient's diagnosis of osteoarthritis, Dr. Tapert started Grant Bowman on intravenous EDTA chelation therapy and a vitamin and mineral supplementation program for its oral chelating effect.

"The patient noticed that his pain had decreased after the seventh IV," Dr. Tapert told us. "He took a one year break from treatment after he had received 25 treatments, since his arthritic pain had completely disappeared. During that year Bowman resumed playing hockey. He gets repeat short courses of chelation therapy (approximately six to eight per year) to maintain his improvement. Playing hockey and tossing 80-pound feed bags are now a routine part of his lifestyle."

Besides the disappearance of arthritis, the patient reports that chelation therapy has helped him in other ways. He has warmer hands and feet and his fingernails and toenails grow faster.

Chelation Therapy for Eye Problems

It's not uncommon for chelation therapy to improve one's eyesight. The treatment has been successfully used to overcome glaucoma, cataracts, diabetic retinopathy, and macular degeneration.

In Encino, California, A. Leonard Klepp, M.D., had under his care Hans Stiglitz, 79 years old, who suffered from dizziness, intermittent claudication (the man could walk only 100 meters at the most before he felt severe calf pain), markedly decreased hearing for which he required a hearing aid, and a long history of high blood pressure. But Stiglitz's most serious health problem was blindness, the result of macular degeneration.

Central vision comes through the macula, the tiny spot in the center of each retina. In macular degeneration, this minute area deteriorates, gradually blurring and eliminating central vision, though leaving most of the peripheral vision intact. The deterioration is most common in the aged, as a result of hardening of the arteries. Thus, macular degeneration is partial or total loss of the sensitive macular area in the retina, which provides sight and color vision. The consequence is a reduced ability to see.

Physical and laboratory examinations of the patient indicated to Dr. Klepp that Stiglitz was an ailing man with some serious health problems. The doctor first met him December 3, 1981, when the full diagnostic workup was conducted. Stiglitz was found to be diabetic with an overly high fasting blood sugar of 174 mg percent.

"His fasting insulin was 45 micro-units per milliliter (ml), with reference normals for this laboratory being 5 to 25. Non-invasive blood flow studies demonstrated aortic occlusion and/or bilateral iliac artery obstruction with openings distally, high left femoral artery obstruction, and small vessel disease of both lower extremities," Dr. Klepp reported. "In the cerebral vascular area, the OCVM [a diagnostic test] showed stenosis [narrowing] of the right carotid [artery] of 48 percent and on the left side 36 percent.

"The patient was seen at Doheny Eye Clinic at the University of Southern California Medical Center, December 10, 1981, and was diagnosed as having macular degeneration, for which nothing could be done," Dr. Klepp wrote to us. Usual treatment for macular degeneration is administration with a focused laser beam. Also, optical devices, known as low-vision aids, may be given for the condition. These are various types of magnifying lenses which provide enlarged images for the victim. But nothing at all had been suggested for Hans Stiglitz by those ophthalmic experts.

Central vision enables one to distinguish detail at close range, as in reading and sewing, and at a distance, as in looking at road signs. Peripheral vision gives perception of your surroundings, including objects and movement not in the direct line of sight. Peripheral vision prevents collisions when walking or driving. If macular degeneration is limited to one eye, the patient can continue to function, but when the disease affects both eyes, as in Stiglitz's case, functioning is altered and the patient must reorient his goals and work.

Doomed to living without any central vision, Hans Stiglitz then returned to Dr. Klepp to find out if this chelating physician might improve the patient's ability to see even though the university ophthalmologists had failed. Dr. Klepp gave the patient 21 chelation treatments. Stiglitz then returned to the University of Southern California Medical Center for another ophthalmic examination on February 9, 1982.

"The ophthalmologists repeated the eye tests and the macula was described as nice and pink," Dr. Klepp said. "In the left eye there was functional improvement three times what it had been before. In the right eye the patient had a 50 to 70 percent improvement. [This book's authors have the actual university eye chart forms and test results for Mr. Stiglitz; the results are exactly as Dr. Klepp has reported.]

"At this point the patient was able to read for the first time in several years, by holding a book up close to his face. He also noticed that his hearing had improved considerably; he was able to hear someone come into the house with his hearing aid removed. His exercise tolerance had also greatly improved," Dr. Klepp said. "This case shows that marked improvement, with objective traditional medical documentation of the progress, was made with this patient, using chelation therapy."

An Alternative to Amputation

H. Richard Casdorph, M.D., Ph.D., of Long Beach, California, currently Assistant Clinical Professor of Medicine at the University of California Medical School, Irvine, California, and a Diplomate in Chelation

Therapy and President of the American College of Advancement in Medicine, and Charles H. Farr, M.D., Ph.D., of Oklahoma City, Oklahoma, former Chairman of the American Board of Chelation Therapy (ABCT) and Diplomate in Chelation Therapy of the ACAM, published a paper in the *Journal of Holistic Medicine* (volume 5, number 1, Spring/Summer 1983) entitled "EDTA Chelation Therapy III: Treatment of Peripheral Arterial Occlusion, an Alternative to Amputation." The paper described four patients, each of whom represented end-stage occlusive peripheral arterial disease with gangrene of the involved extremity. These patients had exhausted all traditional forms of medical treatment, and all had been referred by their individual internists to peripheral vascular surgeons for amputation of their gangrenous legs.

Instead of undergoing surgery, these patients came, in unrelated circumstances, to Drs. Casdorph and Farr, holistic physicians who use alternative methods of healing. The doctors began intravenous EDTA chelation therapy, and the patients' gangrenous conditions were reversed. Healing began, and the patients' once diseased limbs were saved from amputation.

Long-term follow-up by the two chelating physicians, lasting more than a year, indicated that all four patients continued to thrive. Today, each walks on his own feet, their once gangrenous extremities intact and pain free. Before open-minded holistic physicians started using chelation therapy in modern medical practice—and even now when it is scorned by ignorant, misinformed, or negligent traditional physicians who follow the narrowest dictates of organized medicine—the legs of such victims would have been cut off as the only means of saving the patients' lives.

EDTA chelation therapy was the most important therapeutic factor in reversing the natural course of the victims' disease. All four patients had been examined by vascular surgeons who unswervingly recommended amputation. The unfortunate people had exhausted any other available forms of medical and surgical therapy. They were virtually told, "Cut them off!"

These unfortunate people were first seen by Drs. Farr and Casdorph after end-stage complications of ischemia were well established. Ischemia is the cessation of the flow of blood because of a blocked artery. Because ischemia was endangering their lives, the patients had virtually resigned themselves to amputation. Today, however, the blood supply to their limbs is quite adequate, because chelation therapy has unclogged the arteries to these limbs.

Drs. Farr and Casdorph reported: "Basic science studies indicate that EDTA binds and removes ectopic calcium deposits from arterial walls. Moreover, clinical studies have consistently shown improvement of symptoms in both large vessel arterial occlusion and in small vessel disease, with improved blood flow to ischemic areas, following an adequate course of intravenous EDTA chelation therapy."

The doctors concluded: "Clinical evidence reported here and elsewhere supports the use of intravenous EDTA chelation therapy as a safe and effective method of treating occlusive arterial disease of both the medium and small vessel types."

Chelation Treatment Cost and Health Insurance Coverage

The cost of individual EDTA chelation treatments varies in different parts of the country. Medical fees usually depend on at least three factors: the cost of living in the specific local area, the doctor's overhead expenses, and the chelating physician's skill in administering the treatments. The fee per intravenous EDTA infusion ranges from $45 to $100. For instance, as of November 1988, one IV treatment cost $45 in northern Michigan and $65 in western Michigan. Further, fees are $75 in the Orlando, Florida area; $75 in Denver; $85 in Houston; $90 in New York City; $100 in Los Angeles, and $2,500 for a week's in-spa stay in Cottonwood, Alabama. There are additional charges for nutritional supplements, laboratory tests, and other options. The cost of the nutritional supplments (oral chelating agents) is about $50 a week.

EDTA chelation therapy works well for such degenerative diseases as stroke, diabetic retinopathy, and kidney disease. But since it is not recognized by organized medicine for the treatment of these conditions, chelation therapy is not usually covered in health insurance policies.

One possible way to get compensation is, prior to undergoing chelation therapy, to have written permission from the health insurer allowing you to submit your bills for insurance payment. In other words, find out from your insurance carrier to whom you should write for permission to have chelation therapy in order to submit bills for reimbursement. When you receive a positive response to your request, take your treatment. Pay your bills and submit the receipted statements to the responding insurance executive for the cost reimbursement. If the insurance carrier changes its mind about reimbursing your health care costs, send a letter of complaint, accompanied by the executive's permission letter, to the insurance commissioner of your state. Such a procedure may be successful in getting your legitimate reimbursement.

Although health insurance companies routinely pay $35,000 or more for hospital and surgeons' costs for single cases of coronary artery bypass surgery, they usually withhold reimbursement for chelation therapy. Considering that chelation therapy costs about one-tenth of the bypass procedure and carries no associated risk of death, unlike coronary bypass, it would seem illogical that health insurance does not cover chelation therapy. However, check with your health insurance company. Though first denying payment, companies later have been known to send reimbursements to chelation patients who resubmit claims.

EDTA chelation therapy is a standard procedure for lead poisoning and other heavy metal toxicity, acute digitalis intoxication (poisoning from a heart medication), heart arrhythmias, and high calcium levels not controlled by other means. If you have one of these problems, it is likely that you are covered for chelation treatment charges under your health insurance policy. Certainly, testing and office visits to evaluate your medical status—before, during, and after chelation therapy—is considered "routine medical care"; as such, the health insurance company may pay for it, depending on the particular provisions of your policy.

The Health Enhancement Eating Program

The eating plan to complement the physiological benefits of people receiving chelation therapy, is sometimes known as the Health Enhancement Eating Program, which has anti-free-radical and anti-atherosclerotic effects. Dr. Trowbridge modified several successful health menu plans derived from Nathan Pritikin, Michio Kushi, Seale Harris, M.D., and other researchers in nutrition. The Health Enhancement Eating Program works well in conjunction with a routinely performed exercise program and specific daily nutritional supplementation. On the next page are recommended foods and eating guidelines to be used on a regular basis.

Nutritional supplementation helps the chelated patient to maintain himself or herself with concentrated nutrition, which is carried by the body fluids to membranes of the cellular organelles that usually come under attack from free radical exposure. Prescribed in megadoses (higher than recommended by the National Research Council of the National Academy of Sciences), vitamins, minerals, amino acids, enzymes, mucopolysaccharides, herbs, protomorphogens, fiber, hormones, antioxidants, fatty acids, concentrated food molecules, some pharmaceuticals, and other ingredients are often utilized by most holistic physicians for their patients taking chelation therapy.

Nutritional supplementation may be prescribed before, during, and long after chelation therapy is administered. The prescription or dispensation of nutrients by a doctor is standard adjunctive therapy to chelation treatment; the two act synergistically. And as mentioned previously, chelation therapy is part of the entire nutritional approach to holistic healing. Usually nutritional supplementation will be used as a disease-prevention modality between variable intervals of booster injections with intravenous EDTA. The supplments help further the natural chelation processes normally taking place in a person's body. The chelating physician's purpose is to provide his patient's body with whatever additional favorable circumstances are available for the body to metabolize and thrive. Nutritional supplementation is one of the major techniques applied.

Certain guidelines for healthy eating, accompanied by food lists, are given to patients taking chelation therapy at the chelation therapy medical centers worldwide, under the medical direction of nutrition-oriented physicians. The following instructions represent a substantial portion of the Health Enhancement Eating Program.

1. Eat real food at every meal, and snack on vegetables or, occasionally, fruit between meals. Take small bites and chew food thoroughly.

2. Every day eat at least one selection from each of the following vegetable groups: green leafy; red, orange, purple; green; yellow, white; beans, peas; and roots. A portion, or serving, is two or more tablespoons.

3. Eat vegetables raw, juiced at home, or steamed (from 5 to 7 minutes). Vegetable juice should be considered an occasional treat—you need the bulk that comes from the whole food.

4. Have a slice or two of bread or toast with every meal. Be sure it is a hearty whole wheat bread or homemade or health food store whole grain bread. Beware of imitation "whole wheat" breads which are dyed brown. Read labels to assure that you are getting 100 percent whole grain bread. If you have a problem handling sugar (diabetes or hypoglycemia), limit bread to one slice three or four times a day; also limit your consumption of the following vegetables, as they have a higher sugar/starch content: sweet potato, black eye peas, chick peas (garbanzos), kidney beans, pinto beans, navy beans, corn, peas, and lima beans.

5. About six to ten times a week eat one serving from any one of the following protein food groups: red meat, fish/mollusks/crustaceans, poultry, and eggs/egg products. Choose white meat (fish or fowl) or eggs more often than red meat. If you have a problem handling sugar, you may have protein food two or three times a day.

6. Eat meat steamed, broiled, baked, or microwaved —*not* fried, grilled, or boiled. Meat cooked medium or

medium rare is better than well-done. Trim off as much fat as possible and avoid highly marbled meat.

7. Drink at least one 8-ounce glass of water just before or with every meal, between meals, and before or at bedtime.

8. For beverages, drink bottled or mineral water (add fresh-squeezed lime), herbal tea, or plain water. (Use a water purifier if drinking tap water.) If you must have coffee or regular tea, ask your physician for guidelines. (Caffeine-containing beverages are not recommended.)

9. Use sea salt sparingly—or a salt substitute, if you are limiting salt intake. Use unsalted, sweet butter sparingly (instead of margarine); use the following seasonings to add flavor to meat and vegetables; black pepper, caraway, chives, cloves, curry, garlic, ginger, olives, paprika, and sage. Use the following oils with vinegar or lemon juice for salad dressing; virgin olive oil, sesame oil, and other cold-pressed vegetable oils.

10. If you like cold cereal, choose any shredded wheat, puffed wheat or rice, Cheerios™, Grape Nuts Flakes™, or similar low-sugar types. Health food stores and some supermarkets carry steel-cut oats and 7-grain cereals, which are recommended. To add flavor, sprinkle wheat germ on cereal, as well as on other food. (Store the opened jar in the refrigerator to pervent the wheat germ from becoming rancid.)

11. Consume no more than two servings of whole milk products per day (¼ ounce white cheese or ½ pint yogurt constitutes one serving). If you must have milk with cereal, use whole cow's milk (if possible, certified raw milk, rather than homogenized).

12. Eat natural food—no sugar, soda pop, diet soft drinks, candy, cookies, or pastries. After you have eaten healthy for a few weeks, your cravings for sweets will have markedly decreased.

13. Buy fresh meat and vegetables—no packaged, preserved, canned, bottled, or prepared food.

14. Drink alcohol sparingly, if at all. Drink *no more* than one light beer per day, or one small glass of wine (diluted with ice cubes), or one mixed drink, made with water, club soda or diet tonic, lots of ice cubes, and only ½ jigger of liquor on top. Do not stir.

15. At every meal, leave the last bite on your plate—and have no seconds or desserts. If you get hungry later, eat a proper snack to stay in control.

16. Eat only those foods you know are healthy for you—if you have questions or doubts, ask your physician.

17. Whenever possible, center all your meals around fruit and vegetables and other food grown reasonably close to where you live. Choose a broad selection of these, make sure they are as fresh as possible and picked at the peak of their natural ripeness. A home garden in a great idea.

18. Your age, any diseases you may have or have had, your health habits (e.g., smoking), even your sex and occupation will influence your needs for nutrition. Consult your physician for the appropriate adjustments according to these factors.

19. Make sure you take your personal nutritional supplements every day, using the proper program for your personal needs as prescribed by your physician.

The Human Factor in Chelation Patient Care

Martha Nelius, a 66-year-old homemaker from Trinity, a south Texas city over 100 miles from the Houston Health Enhancement Center, consulted Dr. Trowbridge in June 1984 for a number of serious health problems. Mrs. Nelius suffered from severe arteriosclerotic cardiovascular disease after she underwent five coronary artery bypasses in March 1981. She had also had a nine-inch popliteal artery replacement behind her right knee.

"My stomach aorta has been replaced, too," said Mrs. Nelius, "and I've had a carotid artery cleanout on the right side, which eventually clogged again. I knew I still had blood vessel trouble, but I just felt like I didn't want any more surgery."

The medications Mrs. Nelius was taking then included 75 mg. of hydrochlorothiazid, twice a day; 100 mg (20 tablets) of Bufferin™ divided into four doses a day; potassium replacement; and Proloid™, three grains four times a day.

Her history of illness also included several years of high blood pressure, hypercholesterolemia (high serum cholesterol), noted on laboratory studies, and excess total toxic metal burden, predominently nickel, which showed up in the heavy metal screening tests. Mrs. Nelius also had a mild malabsorption pattern, with the result that she was getting insufficient nutrition from the food she ate.

"I had total occlusion in that right leg at my popliteal artery bypass. I could not walk. After taking only a dozen steps, I would be hit with severe leg cramps, [claudication] which forced me to stop and rest, and then walk another dozen steps. I could hardly make it to the local grocery to pick up milk and bread," she said. "I couldn't stand at the sink even to wash our few breakfast dishes. I frequently lost my train of thought— couldn't remember what it was I wanted to say— and I was having trouble with chest pains."

Dr. Trowbridge then started his patient on a series of chelation treatments. Immediately her blood pressure dropped, and it was still normal at the time of this interview, in mid-September 1988.

"After taking chelation therapy I can walk 700 feet without feeling any leg pain. And other amazing things have happened. The new hair on my head is growing in dark brown and thicker, instead of thin and grey. It's like the color my hair was when I was a young girl," Mrs. Nelius said.

"Hair has started to grow again on my arms and legs. Because of poor blood circulation, I hadn't had hair on my legs in years. And before, my toenails had stopped growing; they were hard and crusted. Now they're growing so fast, I have to cut them often and the crusting is soft and easy to clean.

"Previously, my carotid arteries were completely blocked on the right side of my neck and 50 percent closed on the left. Dr. Trowbridge listened to those carotid arteries at my twenty-fourth chelation treatment and found them both fully open and clear," the woman said. The chelating physician thoroughly examines his patients at individually specified intervals of 12 treatments, when he then judges how many more intravenous injections with EDTA may be necessary to eliminate the disease process.

"I'm real proud! I drive myself to Houston from Trinity, which I couldn't do before because my accelerator foot would go to sleep," Martha Nelius concluded. "Now I have no trouble driving. I've come a long way."

According to the physician's report, Mrs. Nelius can get discomfort in her legs with excessive physical activity, and her feet are somewhat cool at times, with occasional cramps when she walks a couple of miles. Otherwise, the woman is remarkably more energetic, never feels chest pain, and is able to perform activities that she could not manage before undergoing chelation therapy.

*   *   *

At age 58, Elmer W. Burgess of Huntsville, Texas, came to the Trowbridge Health Enhancement Center, in February 1984, feeling as if he were going to fall over. The dizzy sensation occurred mostly when he bent down. But he experienced similar symptoms when he looked up or from side to side while walking along the corridors at a Texas State prison facility where he was a guard. Even on land, he felt seasick—as if he were walking the deck of a boat.

Mr. Burgess's unsteadiness was diagnosed as a vertebral basal artery syndrome. The collective causes were obvious to Dr. Trowbridge from his new patient's health history. In 1979, the man had undergone an aorto-femoral bypass operation because of claudication symptoms in his legs. In 1980, Burgess also had five coronary artery bypasses. Then he had a femoral popliteal bypass graft (from the groin to the knee) in 1981 for persistent leg problems. His next operation was a right carotid endarterectomy because of carotid artery atherosclerosis.

Burgess was suffering further with high blood pressure, continuous headaches, frequent colds, coughing, and fungus infection of all the toenails. The poor man was especially terrified of being struck down by a heart attack or stroke or losing a foot or leg. He certainly did have cause for worry.

Prior to starting on chelation therapy, Elmer Burgess was taking a variety of medications including tenormin, 50 mg twice a day; Dyazide™, one tablet four times a day; Motrin™, 400 mg as needed. A screening done under the physician's supervision indicated that the patient had mercury poisoning.

"I was tired a lot, had leg cramps, was just plumb worn out in half a day. Thirty-five thousand dollars worth of open heart surgery didn't seem to have done the job for me," Burgess said. "I knew I had to do something to help myself, and the only thing offered by other doctors and hospitals was more open heart surgery. But two of my friends from Huntsville took courses of chelation therapy. Their physical symptoms disappeared, and both of them felt so much better, I decided I wanted to feel good, too.

"I went through all the pre-chelation diagnostic tests required and then started taking the treatments once a week. I wanted to take three chelations a week, but my work schedule didn't permit it. I've had 26 treatments so far."

Burgess's overall physical wellbeing has improved, his sexual activity has increased tremendously and he is no longer tired during the day. His postural change vertigo (the dizziness) with side to side and upward gaze unsteadiness has gone. He says that his hands and feet stay warmer. His blood pressure is near normal and he needs lower doses of blood pressure medicine than were once necessary.

"Before I received chelation therapy, I used to wear a wool cap to bed, winter and summer, to keep my head warm. Since the sixth chelation treatment, I've thrown away the cap," said Burgess. "Also, my golf game has improved. My mental capacity is more retentive; that state where I could recall an event of several years ago but not something that took place just last week has turned around. My recall is normal.

"It got so that I couldn't walk a block without feeling chest pain. I certainly couldn't climb stairs. On my job we had an upstairs section to the cellblock; let me tell you honestly, I used to avoid whenever possible going up those stairs. I'd hide! Now there's never a problem. I run up stairs whenever I want. I'm addicted to the chelation treatments; I get high off of them.

"In terms of money, chelation therapy is worth it. The $5,000 I'm spending for the pre-chelation testing, my nutritional supplements, and the scheduled 36 chelation treatments compares favorably with the vast sums I've already spent on all that other useless medical care. With chelation treatment, I haven't been cut on; no one is penetrating my body," Burgess pointed out. "I'm really happy to have chelation therapy."

ALABAMA
Birmingham
P. Gus J. Prosch Jr., MD • (205) 823-6180
Huntsville
George Gray, MD • (205) 533-4464
Pat Hamm, MD • (205) 534-8115

ALASKA
Anchorage
F. Russell Manuel, MD • (907) 562-7070
Robert Rowen, MD • (907) 344-7775
Soldotna
Paul G. Isaak, MD • (907) 262-9341
Wasilla
Robert E. Martin, MD • (907) 376-5284

ARIZONA
Cornville
Terry S. Friedmann, MD • (602) 951-2605
Mesa
William W. Halcomb, DO • (602) 832-3014
Dewall J. Hildreth, DO • (602) 390-5737
Parker
S. W. Meyer, DO • (602) 669-8911
Phoenix
Lloyd D. Arnold, DO • (602) 939-8916
Stanley R. Olsztyn, MD • (602) 954-0811
Prescott
Gordon H. Josephs, DO • (602) 778-6169
Scottsdale
Gordon H. Josephs, DO • (602) 998-9232
Tucson
Gordon H. Josephs, DO • (602) 795-5677
Ross S. McConnell, MD • (602) 622-6655

ARKANSAS
Leslie
Melissa Taliaferro, MD • (501) 447-2599
Little Rock
Norbert J. Becquet, MD • (501) 375-4419
John L. Gustavus, MD • (501) 758-9350
Springdale
Doty Murphy III, MD • (501) 756-3251

CALIFORNIA
Auburn
Zane Kime, MD • (916) 823-3421
Bakersfield
Ralph G. Seibly, MD • (805) 873-1000
Campbell
Carol A. Shamlin, MD • (408) 378-7970
Chico
Eva Jalkotzy, MD • (916) 893-3080
Concord
John P. Toth, MD • (415) 682-5660
Covina
James Privitera, MD • (818) 966-1618
El Cajon
William J. Saccoman, MD • (619) 440-3838
El Toro
David A. Steenblock, DO • (714) 770-9616
Encino
Charles Canfield, MD
A. Leonard Klepp, MD • (818) 981-5511
Fresno
David J. Edwards, MD • (209) 251-5066
Grand Terrace
Bruce Halstead, MD • (714) 783-2773
Hollywood
James J. Julian, MD • (213) 467-5555
Huntington Beach
Robert Peterson, DO • (714) 841-6355
Joan M. Resk, DO • (714) 842-2591

La Jolla
Pierre Steiner, MD
Laytonville
Eugene D. Finkle, MD • (707) 984-6151
Long Beach
H. Richard Casdorph, MD, Ph.D., FACAM • (213) 597-8716
Los Altos
Robert F. Cathcart III, MD • (415) 949-2822
Claude Marquette, MD • (415) 964-6700
Los Angeles
Laszlo Belenyessy, MD • (213)822-4614
M. Jahangiri, MD • (213) 587-3218
Monterey
Lon B. Work, MD • (408) 655-0215
Newport Beach
Julian Whitaker, MD • (714) 851-1550
North Highlands
Garry F. Gordon, MD • (916) 348-1011
Oxnard
Mohamed Moharram, MD • (805) 483-2355
David B. Murray, MD • (805) 981-0250
Palm Springs
Sean Degnan, MD • (619) 320-4292
David H. Tang, MD • (619) 320-4292
Petaluma
Mortimer Weiss, MD • (707) 762-5533
Porterville
John B. Park, MD • (209) 781-6224
Rancho Mirage
Charles Farinella, MD • (619) 324-0734
Redding
Bessie J. Tillman, MD • (916) 246-3022
Reseda
Ilona Abraham, MD • (818) 345-8721
Sacramento
Michael Kwiker, DO • (916)489-4400
San Diego
Lawrence H. Taylor, MD • (619) 296-2952
San Francisco
Richard A. Kunin, MD • (415) 346-2500
Paul Lynn, MD • (415) 566-1000
Gary S. Ross, MD • (415)398-0555
San Leandro
Steven H. Gee, MD • (415) 483-5881
San Marcos
William C. Kubitschek, DO • (619) 744-6991
San Rafael
Robert Haskell, MD • (415) 499-9377
Santa Ana
Robert B. Gold, DO • (714) 556-GOLD
Ronald Wempen, MD • (714)546-4325
Santa Barbara
H.J. Hoegerman, MD • (805) 963-1824
Mohamed Moharram, MD • (805) 965-5229
Santa Maria
Donald E. Reiner, MD • (805) 925-0961
Santa Monica
Murray Susser, MD • (213) 453-4424
Seal Beach
Allen Green, MD • (213) 493-4526
Sherman Oaks
Rosa M. Ami Belli, MD
Smith River
James D. Schuler, MD • (707) 487-3405
Stanton
William J. Goldwag, MD • (714) 827-5180
Studio City
Charles E. Law Jr., MD • (818) 761-1661
Torrance
Anita Millen, MD • (213) 320-1132

Van Nuys
Frank Mosler, MD • (818) 785-7425
Walnut Creek
Alan Shifman Charles, MD • (415) 937-3331

COLORADO
Boulder
Barbara Phillips, MD • (303) 449-3112
Colorado Springs
Sandra Denton, MD • (719) 548-1600
James R. Fish, MD • (719) 471-2273
George Juetersonke, DO • (719) 596-9040
Englewood
John H. Altshuler, MD • (303) 740-7771
Grand Junction
William L. Reed, MD • (303) 241-3631
Wheat Ridge
William Doell, DO • (303) 422-0585

CONNECTICUT
Torrington
Jerrold N. Finnie, MD • (203) 489-8977

DISTRICT OF COLUMBIA
Washington
Paul Beals, MD • (202) 223-5714
George H. Mitchell, MD • (202) 265-4111

FLORIDA
Atlantic Beach
Richard Worsham, MD
Boca Raton
Narinder Singh Parhar, MD • (407) 479-3200
Bradenton
Eteri Melnikov, MD • (813) 748-7943
Crystal River
Carlos F. Gonzalez, MD • (904)795-4711
Delray Beach
Moyses Chaplik, MD • (407) 499-8200
Fort Myers
Gary L. Pynckel, DO • (813) 278-3377
Holly Hill
Sam D. Matheny, DO • (904) 672-2111
Hollywood
Herbert Pardell, DO • (305) 989-5558
Ricardo Sabates, MD • (305) 989-5558
Jupiter
Neil Ahner, MD • (407) 744-0077
Lakeland
Harold Robinson, MD • (813) 646-5088
Lauderhill
Herbert R. Slavin, MD • (305) 748-4991
Maitland
Joya Lynn Schoen, MD • (407) 644-2729
Miami
Joseph G. Godorov, DO • (305) 595-0671
North Lauderdale
Narinder Singh Parhar, MD • (305) 978-6604
North Miami Beach
Martin Dayton, DO • (305) 931-8484
Ocala
George Graves, DO • (904) 236-2525 or
(904) 732-3633
Orlando
James Parsons, MD • (407) 870-5005
Palm Bay
Neil Ahner, MD • (407) 729-8581
Pensacola
Ward Dean, MD • (904) 484-0595
Pompano Beach
Dan C. Roehm, MD • (305) 977-3700
Port Canaveral
James Parsons, MD • (407) 784-2102

Royal Palm Beach
Domenico Caporusso, MD • (407) 793-7548
St. Petersburg
Ray Wunderlich Jr., MD • (813) 822-3612
Tampa
Eugene H. Lee, MD • (813) 251-3089
Venice
Thomas McNaughton, MD • (813) 484-2167
Wauchula
Alfred S. Massam, MD • (813) 773-6668
Winter Park
James M. Parsons, MD • (407) 628-3399
Robert Rogers, MD • (407) 679-1111

GEORGIA
Atlanta
David Epstein, DO • (404) 525-7333
Milton Fried, MD • (404) 451-4857
Camilla
Oliver L. Gunter, MD • (912) 336-7343
Norcross
Bernard Mlaver, MD • (404) 448-4535
Warner Robins
Terril J. Schneider, MD • (912) 929-1027

HAWAII
Kailua-Kona
Clifton Arrington, MD • (808) 322-9400

IDAHO
Coeur d'Alene
Charles T. McGee, MD • (208) 664-1478
Nampa
John O. Boxall, MD • (208) 466-3517
Sandpoint
K. Peter McCallum, MD • (208) 263-5456

ILLINOIS
Arlington Heights
Terrill K. Haws, DO • (708) 577-9451
William Mauer, DO, FACAM • (708) 255-8988
Aurora
Thomas Hesselink, MD • (708) 844-0011
Belvidere
M. Paul Dommers, MD • (815) 544-3112
Chicago
Charles Kaplan, MD • (312) 348-2882
Razvan Rentea, MD • (312) 549-0101
Downers Grove
Guillermo Justiniano, MD • (708) 964-8083
Geneva
Richard E. Hrdlicka, MD • (708) 232-1900
Glen Ellyn
Robert S. Waters, MD • (708) 790-8100
Homewood
Frederick Weiss, MD
Metamora
S.K. Elsasser, DO, FACAM • (309) 367-2321
Moline
Terry W. Love, DO • (309) 764-2900
Oak Park
Paul J. Dunn, MD • (708) 383-3800
Ottawa
Terry W. Love, DO • (815) 434-1977
Woodstock
John R. Tambone, MD • (815) 338-2345

INDIANA
Clarksville
George Wolverton, MD • (812) 282-4309
Evansville
Harold T. Sparks, DO • (812) 479-8228
Highland
Cal Streeter, DO • (219) 924-2410

Indianapolis
David A. Darbro, MD • (317) 787-7221
Mooresville
Norman E. Whitney, DO • (317) 831-3352
South Bend
David E. Turfler, DO • (219) 233-3840

IOWA
Davenport
David P. Nebbeling, DO • (319) 391-0321

KANSAS
Andover
Stevens B. Acker, MD • (316) 733-4494
Garden City
Terry Hunsberger, DO • (316) 275-7128
Hays
Roy N. Neil, MD • (913) 628-8341
Kansas City
John Gamble, Jr., DO • (913) 321-1140

KENTUCKY
Bowling Green
John C. Tapp, MD • (502) 781-1483
Louisville
Kirk Morgan, MD • (502) 228-0156
Nicholasville
Walt Stoll, MD • (606) 233-4273
Somerset
Stephen S. Kiteck, MD • (606) 678-5137

LOUISIANNA
Baton Rouge
Steve Kuplesky, MD
Chalmette
Saroj T. Tampira, MD • (504) 277-8991
Mandeville
Roy M. Montalbano, MD • (504) 626-1985
Newellton
Joseph R. Whitaker, MD • (318) 467-5131
New Iberia
Adonis J. Domingue, MD • (318) 365-2196
New Orleans
James P. Carter, MD • (504) 588-5136
Shreveport
R. Denman Crow, MD • (318) 221-1569

MAINE
Van Buren
Joseph Cyr, MD • (207) 868-5273

MARYLAND
Laurel
Paul V. Beals, MD • (301) 490-9911

MASSACHUSETTS
Barnstable
Richard H. Cohen, MD • (508) 362-9797
Michael Janson, MD • (508) 362-4343
Cambridge
Michael Janson, MD • (617) 661-6225
Hanover
Richard Cohen, MD • (617) 829-9281
Holden
N. Thomas La Cava, MD • (508) 829-5321
Long Meadow
Richard Cohen, MD • (413) 567-2400
Newton Centre
Carol Englender, MD • (617) 965-7770

MICHIGAN
Atlanta
Leo Modzinski, DO,MD • (517) 785-4254
Bay City
Doyle B. Hill, DO • (517) 686-5200

Detroit
Richard E. Tapert, DO • (313) 885-5405
John R. Verbovsky, DO • (313) 366-2050
Farmington Hills
Paul A. Parente, DO • (313) 626-7544
Paul A. Parente, DO • (313) 626-9690
Albert J. Scarchilli, DO • (313) 626-7544
Albert J. Scarchilli, DO • (313) 626-9690
Flint
William M. Bernard, DO • (313) 733-3140
Kenneth Ganapini, DO • (313) 733-3140
Grand Haven
E. Duane Powers, DO
Grand Rapids
Grant Born, DO • (616) 455-3550
Linden
Marvin D. Penwell, DO • (313) 735-7809
Pontiac
Vahagn Agbabian, DO • (313) 334-2424

MINNESOTA
Minneapolis
Jean R. Eckerly, MD • (612) 593-9458
Keith J. Carlson, MD • (507) 247-5921

MISSISSIPPI
Coldwater
Pravinchandra Patel, MD • (601) 622-7011
Columbus
James H. Sams, MD • (601) 327-8701
Ocean Springs
James H. Waddell, MD • (601) 875-5505
Shelby
Robert Hollingsworth, MD • (601) 398-5106

MISSOURI
Festus
John T. Schwent, DO • (314) 937-8688
Independence
James E. Swann, DO • (816) 833-3366
Kansas City
Edward W. McDonagh, DO, FACAM • (816) 453-5940
James Rowland, DO • (816) 361-4077
Charles Rudolph, DO,Ph.D, FACAM • (816) 453-5940
Springfield
William C. Sunderwirth, DO • (417) 869-6260
St. Louis
Harvey Walker Jr., MD, Ph.D, FACAM • (314) 721-7227
Stockton
William C. Sunderwirth, DO • (417) 276-3221
Sullivan
Ronald H. Scott, DO • (314) 468-4932
Union
Clinton C. Hayes, DO • (314) 583-8911

NEBRASKA
Ord
Otis W. Miller, MD • (308) 728-3251

NEVADA
Incline Village
W. Douglas Brodie, MD • (702) 832-7001
Las Vegas
Ji-Zhou (Jos.) Kang, MD • (702) 798-2992
Robert D. Milne, MD • (702) 385-1999
Terry Pfau, DO • (702) 385-1999
Dan F. Royal, DO (702) 732-1400
Robert Vance, DO • (702) 385-7771
Reno
Michael L. Gerber, MD • (702) 826-1900
Donald E. Soli, MD • (702) 786-7101
Yiwen Y. Tang, MD • (702) 826-9500

NEW JERSEY
Bloomfield
Majid Ali, MD • (201) 743-1151
Cherry Hill
Allan Magaziner, DO • (609) 424-8222
Edison
C. Y. Lee, MD • (908) 738-9220
Ralph Lev, MD, MS • (908) 738-9220
Richard B. Menashe, DO • (908) 906-8866
Paramus
Leonard J. Gorkun, MD • (201) 967-5081
West Orange
Faina Munits, MD • (201) 736-3743

NEW MEXICO
Albuquerque
Ralph J. Luciani, DO • (505) 888-5995
Gerald Parker, DO • (505) 884-3506
John T. Taylor, DO • (505) 884-3506
Roswell
Annette Stoesser, MD • (505) 623-2444

NEW YORK
Brooklyn
Michael Teplitsky, MD • (718) 769-0997
Pavel Yutsis, MD • (718) 234-0500
East Meadow
Christopher Calapai, DO • (516) 794-0404
Falconer
Reino Hill, MD • (716) 665-3505
Huntington
Serafina Corsello, MD, FACAM • (516) 271-0222
Kingspoint
Mary F. Di Rico, MD • (516) 466-3407
Lawrence
Mitchell Kurk, MD • (516) 239-5540
New York
Robert C. Atkins, MD • (212) 758-2110
Serafina Corsello, MD, FACAM • (212) 399-0222
Ronald Hoffman, MD • (212) 779-1744
Richard Izquierdo, MD • (212) 589-4541
Warren M. Levin, MD • (212) 696-1900
Niagara Falls
Paul Cutler, MD, FACAM • (716) 284-5140
Orangeburg
Neil L. Block, MD • (914) 359-3300
Plattsburgh
Driss Hassam, MD • (518) 561-2023
Rhinebeck
Kenneth A. Bock, MD • (914) 876-7082
Suffern
Michael B. Schachter, MD, FACAM • (914) 368-4700
Watervliet
Rodolfo T. Sy, MD • (518) 273-1325
Westbury
Savely Yurkovsky, MD • (516) 333-2929

NORTH CAROLINA
Aberdeen
Keith E. Johnson, MD • (919) 281-5122
Leicester
John L. Laird, MD • (704) 683-3101
Statesville
John L. Laird, MD • (704) 876-1617 or (800) 445-4762

NORTH DAKOTA
Grand Forks
Richard H. Leigh, MD • (701) 775-5527

Minot
Brian E. Briggs, MD • (701) 838-6011

OHIO
Akron
Josephine Aronica, MD • (216) 867-7361
Bluffton
L. Terry Chappell, MD, FACAM • (419) 358-4627
Canton
Jack E. Slingluff, DO • (216) 494-8641
Cleveland
John M. Baron, DO • (216) 642-0082
James P. Frackelton, MD, FACAM • (216) 835-0104
Derrick Lonsdale, MD, FACAM • (216) 835-0104
Douglas Weeks, MD • (216) 835-0104
Columbus
Robert R. Hershner, DO • (614) 253-8733
Seldon R. Nelson, MD • (614) 761-0555
Dayton
David D. Goldberg, DO • (513) 277-1722
Paulding
Don K. Snyder, MD • (419) 399-2045
Youngstown
James Ventresco Jr., DO • (216) 792-2349

OKLAHOMA
Jenks
Leon Anderson, DO • (918) 299-5039
Oklahoma City
Charles H. Farr, MD, Ph.D • (405) 632-8868
Charles D .Taylor, MD • (405) 525-7751

OREGON
Eugene
John Gambee, MD • (503) 686-2536
Grants Pass
James Fitzsimmons Jr., MD • (503) 474-2166
Salem
Terence Howe Young, MD • (503) 371-1558

PENNSYLVANIA
Allentown
Robert H. Schmidt, DO • (215) 437-1959
D. Erik Von Kiel, DO • (215) 776-7639
Bangor
Francis J. Cinelli, DO • (215) 588-4502
Elizabethtown
Dennis L. Gilbert, DO • (717) 367-1345
Fountainville
Harold H. Byer, MD, PhD • (215) 348-0443
Greensburg
Ralph A. Miranda, MD • (412) 838-7632
Hazleton
Arthur L. Koch, DO • (717) 455-4747
Macungie
D. Erik Von Kiel, DO • (215) 967-5503
Mertztown
Conrad G. Maulfair Jr., DO, FACAM • (215) 682-2104
Mt. Pleasant
Mamduh El-Attrache, MD • (412) 547-3576
North Versailles
Mamduh El-Attrache, MD • (412) 673-3900
Philadelphia
Frederick Burton, MD • (215) 844-4660
P. Jayalakshmi, MD • (215) 473-4226
K. R. Sampathachar, MD • (215) 473-4226
Lance Wright, MD • (215) 387-1200
Pittsburgh
Howard T. Lewis, MD • (412) 531-1222

Quakertown
Harold Buttram, MD • (215) 536-1890

SOUTH CAROLINA
Columbia
Theodore C. Rozema, MD • (803) 796-1702
Landrum
Theodore C. Rozema, MD • (803) 457-4141
(800) 922-5821 (SC) (800) 992-8350 (NAT)

TENNESSEE
Jackson
S. Marshall Fram, MD
Morristown
Donald Thompson, MD • (615) 581-6367

TEXAS
Abilene
William Irby Fox, MD • (915) 672-7863
Alamo
Herbert Carr, DO • (512) 787-6668
Amarillo
Gerald Parker, DO • (806) 355-8263
John T. Taylor, DO • (806) 355-8263
Austin
Vladimir Rizov, MD • (512) 451-8149
Dallas
Michael G. Samuels, DO • (214) 991-3977
J. Robert Winslow, DO • (214) 243-7711
J. Robert Winslow, DO • (214) 241-4614
El Paso
Edward J. Ettl, MD • (915) 566-9361
Francisco Soto, MD • (915) 534-0272
Houston
Robert Battle, MD • (713) 932-0552
Jerome L. Borochoff, MD • (713) 461-7517
Luis E. Guerrero, MD • (713) 789-0133
Paul McGuff, MD • (713) 780-7019
Carlos E. Nossa, MD • (713) 783-6009
Humble
John Parks Trowbridge, MD, FACAM • (713) 540-2329
Kirbyville
John L. Sessions, DO • (409) 423-2166
La Porte
Ronald M. Davis, MD • (713) 470-2930
San Antonio
Jim P. Archer, DO • (512) 694-4091
Wichita Falls
Thomas R. Humphrey, MD • (817) 766-4329

UTAH
Provo
Dennis Harper, DO • (801) 373-8500

VIRGINIA
Annandale
Sohini Patel, MD • (703) 941-3606
Hinton
Harold Huffman, MD • (703) 867-5242
Midlothian
Peter C. Gent, DO • (804) 744-3551
Norfolk
Vincent Speckhart, MD • (804) 622-0014
Trout Dale
E. M. Cranton, MD, FACAM • (703) 677-3631

WASHINGTON
Bellingham
Robert Kimmel, MD • (206) 734-3250
Kent
Jonathan Wright, MD • (206) 631-8920
Kirkland
Jonathan Collin, MD • (206) 820-0547
Port Townsend
Jonathan Collin, MD • (206) 385-4555
Spokane
Burton B. Hart, DO • (509) 927-9922
Vancouver
Richard P. Huemer, MD • (206) 253-4445
Yakima
Murray L. Black, DO • (509) 966-1780
Richard Wilkinson, MD • (509) 453-5506
Yelm
Elmer Cranton, MD, FACAM • (206) 894-3548

WEST VIRGINIA
Beckley
Prudencio Corro, MD • (304) 252-0775
Charleston
Steve M. Zekan, MD • (304) 343-7559
Follansbee
Albert Molisky, DO • (304) 527-1626
Iaeger
Ebb K. Whitley Jr., MD • (304) 938-5357
Midway
Michael Kostenko, DO • (304) 683-3251

WISCONSIN
Green Bay
Eleazar M. Kadile, MD • (414) 468-9442
Lake Geneva
Rathna Alwa, MD • (414) 248-1430
Milwaukee
William J. Faber, DO • (414) 464-7680
Thomas Hessellink, MD • (414) 259-1350
Robert R. Stocker, DO • (414) 258-6282
Wisconsin Dells
Robert S. Waters, MD • (608) 254-7178

1992 MEMBERSHIP ROSTER (INTERNATIONAL)
AMERICAN COLLEGE OF ADVANCEMENT IN MEDICINE

AUSTRALIA
Donvale, Victoria
R.B. Allen, MD • 011-613-842-6472
Gosford, N.S.W.
Heather M. Bassett, MD • (043) 24 7388

BELGIUM
Antwerpen
Didier Langouche, MD • 32-03-2250313
Ghent
Michel De Meyer, MD • 091-22-33-42
St. Niklaasa
A. De Bruyne, MD • 011-32-031-7774150

BRAZIL
Amazonas
Fernando de Souza, MD • 011-55-92-2367733
Curitiba
Oslim Malina, MD • 011-41-2524395
Florianopolis
Jose P. Figueredo, MD • 011-482-22-4960
Osorio-RS
Jose Valdai de Souza, MD • 011-55-51-6631269
Pelotas-RS
Antonio C. Fernandes, MD • 011-55-53-2224699

BRAZIL ▬

Porto Alegre
Moyses Hodara, MD • 011-55-51-2243557
Carlos J. P. de Sa, MD • 011-55-51-2334832
Rio Preto
A.O. Passos Correa, MD • 011-55-17-2334455
Sao Paulo
Guilherme Deucher, MD • 011-55-11-5719100
Fernando L. Flaquer, MD • 011-55-2112019
Sergio Vaisman, MD • 011-55-11-2108210

CANADA
- British Columbia -
Argenta
Robert Sweeney, MD • (604) 366-4265
Errington
George Barber, MD • (604) 248-8956
Kelowna
Alex A. Neil, MD • (604) 765-4117
Vancouver
Kevin R. Nolan, MD • (604) 736-8338
Saul Pilar, MD • (604) 736-8338
Donald W. Stewart, MC • (604) 732-1348
Zigurts Strauts, MD • (604) 736-1105
Victoria
Deanne Roberts, MD • (604) 370-4377
- Manitoba -
Winnepeg
Howard N. Reed, MD • (204) 957-1900
- Ontario -
Blythe
Richard W. Street, MD • (519) 523-4433
Sarnia
Nazer Vellani, MD • (519) 344-6171
Smiths Falls
Clare Minielly, MD • (613) 283-7703
Willowdale
Paul Cutler, MD, FACAM • (416) 733-3151

DENMARK
Aarhus
Kurt Christensen, MD • 06-126141
Bruce P. Kyle, MD • 86-293550
Humlebaek
Joergen Rugaard, MD
Lyngby
Claus Hancke, MD • 45 42 88 09 00
Skodsborg
Bo Mogelvang, MD • 011-4542803200
Niels Ove Pedersen, MD • 011-4542803200
Vejle
Knut T. Flytlie, MD • 011-4575820346
Virum
Pierre Eggers-Lura, MD • 011-4502863961

DOMINICAN REPUBLIC
Santo Domingo
Antonio Pannocchia, MD • 565-3259

EGYPT
Cairo
Elham G. Behery, MD • 011-202-3484517

ENGLAND
Kent
F. Schellander, MD • 011-44-892-543536
West Sussex
Simi Khanna, MD • 011-44-342-324984

FRANCE
Paris
Bruno Crussol, MD • 011-33-1-47551919
Paul Musarella, MD • 011-33-1-45621938

GERMANY
Bad Fussing
Karl Heinz Caspers, MD • 011-49-8531-21001
or 011-49-8531-21004
Bad Steben
Helmut Keller, MD • 011-49-9288-5166
Rattach-Egern
Claus Martin, MD • 011-49-8022-6415
Werne
Jens-Ruediger Collatz, MD • 02389-3883

INDONESIA
Bandung
Benj. Widjajakusuma, MD • (022) 615277
Jakarta
Maimunah Affandi, MD • (021) 716927
Adjit Singh Gill, MD • (021) 357359
Yahya Kisyanto, MD • (021) 334636

ITALY
Michele Ballo, MD • 91-580301

MALAYSIA
Mohamed S.A. Ishak, MD • 06-235878/06-239396

MEXICO
Chihuahua
H. Berlanga Reyes, MD • (95) 141-3-92-71 or
(95) 141-3-92-75
Guadalajara, Jalisco
Eleazar A. Carrasco, MD • 25-16-55
F. Navares Merino, MD • (36) 16-88-70
Juarez, Chih.
H. Berlanga Reyes, MD • 13-80-23
Francisco Soto, MD • 011-52-16-162-601
Matamoros, Tamp.
Frank Morales Sr., MD • 3-31-07
Tijuana
Francisco Rique, MD • (706) 681-3171
Rodrigo Rodriguez, MD • (706) 681-3171
Roberto Tapia, MD • (706) 681-3171
Torreon, Coahuila
Carlos Lopez Moreno, MD • 011-52-17-138140

NETHERLANDS
Bilthoven
C.J.M. Broekhuyse, MD • 011-30-250774
Etten-Leur
Peter Zeegers, MD • 011-31-1608-17127
Haarlem
Eduard Schweden, MD • 011-31-23-328833
Dirk van Lith, MD • 011-31-23328833
Leende
Peter van der Schaar, MD • 011-31-4959-2232
Marc Verheyen, MD • 011-31-49592232
Loernersloot
A. Verbon, MD • 011-31-2949-1289
Maastricht
Rob van Zandvoort, MD • 011-31-4362-3474
Oudenbosch
E. T. Oei, MD • 011-31-1652-17455
Rotterdam
Robert T.H.K. Trossel, MD • 01131 10 4126362/
4147633
Utrecht
P.J.C. Riethoven, MD • 030-518951
Velp
J. H. Leenders, MD • 31-085-642742

NETHERLANDS-ANTILLES
Aruba
Adhemar E. Hart, MD • 011-297-8-27263

NETHERLANDS-ANTILLES ▬

St. Maarten
Dirk van Lith, MD • 011-5995-53097
Robert T.H.K. Trossel, MD • 011-5995-53097

NEW ZEALAND
Auckland
Maurice B. Archer, DO • 011-64-9-303-2847
R.H. Bundellu, MD • 011-64-9-2746701
Christchurch
Robert Blackmore, MD • (03) 853-015
Hamilton
William J. Reeder, MD • (071) 78425
Masterton
T. J. Baily Gibson, MD • (059) 81-250
New Lynn
Raymond Ramirez, MD • (09) 872-200
Napier
Tony Edwards, MD • (070) 354-696
Oxford, No. Canterbury
Ted Walford, MD (075) 86-808
Taurange
Michael E. Godfrey, MD • (075) 782-362

PHILIPPINES
Manila
Rosa M. Ami Belli, MD • 50-03-23
Leonides Lerma, MD • 57-59-11

Corazon Macawili-Yu, MD • 50-03-23
Remedios L. Reynoso, MD • 50-03-23

PUERTO RICO
Cidra
Pedro Rivera, MD • (809) 732-8053
Santurce
Pedro Zayas, MD • (809) 727-1105

SPAIN
Malaga
Henning Munksnaes, MD • 011-34-52-493358

SWITZERLAND
Geneva
Robert Tissot, MD • (22) 498875
Montreux
Claude Rossel, MD, PhD • 21-6351-01
Netstal (Glarus)
Walter Blumer, MD • 058-61-28-46

TAIWAN (R.O.C.)
Taipei
Paul Lin, MD • (02) 507-2222 (Taipei) Ext. 1003
Yeh-Sung Lin, MD • 886-2-507-8349

WEST INDES
Jamaica
H. Marco Brown, MD • 011-809-952-3454

Reprinted from the 1992 Membership Roster of the American College of
Advancement in Medicine (used with permission).

SMART **N**UTRIENTS
A Guide to Nutrients That Can Enhance Intelligence and Reverse Senility
by Dr. Abram Hoffer and Dr. Morton Walker

Issued as a quality paperback ISBN # 0-89529-562-8 by the Avery Publishing
Group, Inc. under its new imprint, "A Dr. Morton Walker Book," 225 pages,
US$9.95 + US$3.05 mail order postage and handling = US$13.00 per book

• This book proves "senile" symptoms are unrelated to aging
-- and may even be caused by well-meaning treatment.
• The stresses of modern life, the popularity of junk foods,
and the pervasiveness of pollutants in the environment have
more to do with senility than the simple fact of growing old.
• Nutritional therapy and the administration of vitamins,
minerals, and other nutrients have halted, corrected or
reversed senility in thousands of patients all over the world.
• Here you will learn the formerly unsuspected and
invaluable properties of certain nutritional supplements.
• Basically, you'll discover that *lower intelligence* and
genuine senility are both forms of nutrient malnutrition.
• Described are the physical and mental changes
contributing to senility, how they get produced, and why
innovative treatment explained here corrects the condition.
• The controversial drug GH3 which restores youthfulness
and reverses the effects of aging is discussed by the authors.

PROVIDED in **S**mart **N**utrients The full nutrition plan, complete lists of nutrients to
avoid senility and raise intelligence, plus the food sources from which to get them.

ORDER FORM: Mail with correct payment to FREELANCE COMMUNICATIONS
484 High Ridge Road, Stamford, Connecticut 06905-3020; Phone (203) 322-1551
SMART **N**UTRIENTS,, A Guide to Nutrients that Enhance Intelligence and Reverse Senility

1 book = US$9.95 + US$3.05 postage & handling = US$13.00, sent Fourth class mail
(To receive the book by US Priority Mail, add US$3.05 more for special handling)
2 - 24 books, deduct 20% = US$7.97 per book + US$2.05 per book for postage & handling
25 - 99 books, deduct 30% = US$6.97 per book + US$1.05 per book for postage & handling
100 books or more, deduct 40% = US$5.97 per book = $0.55 per book for postage & handling

----

My payment to FREELANCE COMMUNICATIONS, 484 High Ridge Rd., Stamford, CT 06905
(Check or Money Order accepted, and no charge accounts, no returns, no refunds granted)

of US$_____is enclosed for a_____percent discount on _____copies of
SMART **N**UTRIENTS by Dr. Abram Hoffer and Dr. Morton Walker

My Name_____

Address_____

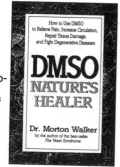

The Chelation Answer

By Dr. Morton Walker

How to Prevent Hardening of the Arteries and Rejuvenate Your Cardiovascular Syste

This book contains the full protocol of treatment administration followed by chelating physicians. Written in easy-read language, it is an ideal text to offer prospective patients in order to have them understand the mechanism chelation therapy and what beneficial effects take place inside the body.

The Chelation Answer explains:

Who is a candidate for treatment
Disease conditions that respond to chelation therapy
Any possible side effects
Contraindications
Insurance reimbursement
Food and Drug Administration rulings on the treatment
American Medical Association opinion,
Related political ramifications
Malpractice committed by physicians who don't offer chelation therapy
Chelation detoxification of the recipient's entire body

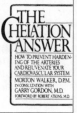

**In brief, this book is a marvelous educational tool for
the chelating physician to offer his or her patients**

Indexed, this 6" x 9" hardcover book, originally published by M. Evans, has 256 pages with a full bibliography.
Reversion of rights are to the author, Dr. Morton Walker. *The Chelation Answer* retails at
$16.95 plus $3.05 for postage by fourth class mail (US$20) (1st class mail delivery or UPS, $3.00 additional charge)

The Chelation Way

By Dr. Morton Walker

The Complete Book of Chelation Therapy

How to Use Chelation Therapy to Reverse Hardening
of the Arteries and Prevent Degenerative Diseases

*The Chelation Way presents information on
intravenous and oral chelation therapy that controls:*

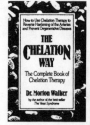

hardened arteries	glaucoma	Lou Gehrig's disease	Alzheimer's disease
angina pectoris	cataracts	Parkinson's disease	Raynaud's disease
heart attack	diabetic retinopathy	high blood pressure	sickle cell anemia
heart arrhythmias	macular degeneration	high blood cholesterol	digitalis intoxication
lupus erythematosus	cancer	osteoporosis	schizophrenia
arthritis	kidney disease	radiation toxicity	varicose veins
diabetes	liver disease	heavy metal toxicity	
gangrene	multiple sclerosis	senility	*and ...*
stroke			
senility			
impotence			

*other degenerative diseases occurring from
impaired blood flow anywhere in the human body*

But intravenous chelation treatments aren't always available, therefore, the second half of *The Chelation Way* provid
the only complete description ever written of oral chelating agents for getting self-help at home. It tells you what t
oral chelating agents are, their full formulations, where to find them, what dosage to take, and what it costs for oral
administered chelating nutrients and drugs that are legal and readily accessible. The American College of Advanceme
in Medicine has furnished its membership list and permission for Dr. Morton Walker to identify all known trained a
qualified chelating physicians in the world, including their names, addresses, and telephone numbers.

Published by Avery Publishing Group, Inc., this quality paperback is 278 pages, 6" x 9" format and is only
$12.95 plus $3.05 for postage (US$16) (1st class delivery or UPS, $3.00 additional charge)

To order either of these fine books, please send your payment including postage to:
FREELANCE COMMUNICATIONS, 484 High Ridge Road, Stamford, Connecticut 06905-3095
Please call (203)322-1551 or fax (203)322-4656 for substantial discounts on bulk orders